AF446815

BRUNNER · KRAUSE · ROTHAUGE · WEIDNER

Chronic Prostatitis

Chronic Prostatitis

Clinical, Microbiological, Cytological and Immunological Aspects of Inflammation

Edited by

H. Brunner, Wuppertal
W. Krause, Marburg
C. F. Rothauge, Gießen
W. Weidner, Gießen

With 52 Figures and 59 Tables

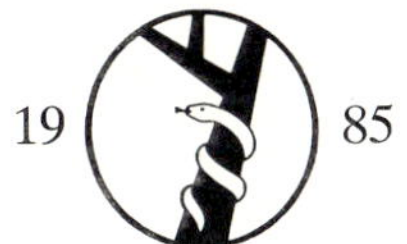

19 85

F. K. SCHATTAUER VERLAG · STUTTGART – NEW YORK

CIP-Kurztitelaufnahme der Deutschen Bibliothek

Deutsche Bibliothek Cataloguing-in-Publication Data

Chronic prostatitis : clin., microbiolog.,
cytolog. and immunolog. aspects of inflammation
/ ed. by H. Brunner ... − Stuttgart ; New York :
Schattauer, 1985.
  ISBN 3-7945-0978-1
NE: Brunner, Helmut [Hrsg.]

Composing, printing and binding: Allgäuer Zeitungsverlag GmbH, Kempten

ISBN 3-7945-0978-1

Preface

Although numerous publications already summarize most aspects of genital tract infections, we thought it might be rewarding to edit a book on chronic prostatitis, because a review on this disease in English does to the best of our knowledge not exist as yet. Such a monograph could be of special interest, because chronic prostatitis is a frequently occurring disease which afflicts increasing numbers of patients and concerns several medical disciplines. Since the etiology and the pathogenesis of chronic prostatitis is poorly understood at the present time and consequently the therapy is unsatisfactory, we thought, that a summary of present knowledge on the clinical, the microbiological and the immunological aspects of this disease might stimulate further research on the multifactorial problems concerned with this syndrome.

The patients present with various symptoms to the physician who is frequently confronted with the problem that his patient has already consulted one or several doctors previously without permanent cure. Since the etiology of this disease is manifold, special diagnostic procedures have been developed, which are laborious and must include various microbiological and immunological techniques. It is therefore essential that a team of experts in various subjects of modern medicine (urologists, andrologist, gynecologists, medical microbiologists and immunologists) work closely together to provide optimal diagnosis and treatment, avoiding that the patient becomes a "prostate-cripple".

This book reviews the various aspects of chronic prostatitis in articles written by specialists with much expertise in the individual area. The editors would be satisfied if this monograph helps the practicing physician and the diagnostic laboratory and, in addition, would stimulate further research on this important medical problem.

The editors would like to gratefully acknowledge the continued efforts and assistance of Prof. Dr. med. Dr. med. h.c. P. Matis and Mrs. G. Stapelberg of the F. K. Schattauer Verlag in the production of this volume.

H. Brunner
W. Krause
C. F. Rothauge
W. Weidner

Contents

List of Contributors

ANDERSON, Dr. R. U.
  Division of Urology, Dept. of Surgery, Stanford University School of Medicine, Stanford, Calif. 94305/USA

ARENS, Dr. M.
  Institut für Hygiene und Infektionskrankheiten der Tiere, Frankfurter Straße 89, D−6300 Gießen/FRG

BAERT, Dr. L.
  Dept. of Urology, O. L. Vrouw Hospital, B−8500 Kortrijk/Belgium (Present address: De Haernelaan, 58, B−8500 Kortrijk)

BALERNA, Dr. M.
  Abteilung gynäkologische Endokrinologie am Krankenhaus "La Carita", CH−6600 Locarno/Switzerland

BAUER, Dr. H. W.
  Urologische Klinik und Poliklinik der Universität München, Klinikum Großhadern, Marchioninistraße 15, D−8000 München 70/FRG

BECKER, H. C.
  Urologische Universitätsklinik, Klinikstraße 37a, D−6300 Gießen/FRG

BERETTA, Dr. G.
  Provinzhospital Magenta, Arbeitsgruppe Andrologie, Abteilung Urologie, Corso Cristoforo Colombo 8, I−20144 Mailand/Italy

BLACKLOCK, Dr. N. J.
  Dept. of Urology, University Hospital South Manchester, Well Lane, West Didsbury, Manchester M 20 BLR/GB

BLENK, Dr. H.
  Institut für Wehrmedizin und Hygiene, Ernst-Rodenwaldt-Institut, Viktoriastraße 11−13, D−5400 Koblenz/FRG

BRUNNER, Prof. Dr. H.
  Bayer AG, Pharma-Forschungszentrum, Institut für Chemotherapie, Postfach 101709, D−5600 Wuppertal 1/FRG

CAMPANA, Dr. A.
  Abteilung gynäkologische Endokrinologie am Krankenhaus "La Carita", CH−6600 Locarno/Switzerland

COLPI, Dr. G. M.
  Provinzhospital Magenta, Arbeitsgruppe Andrologie, Abteilung Urologie, Corso Cristoforo Colombo 8, I−20144 Mailand/Italy

DEBRUYNE, Dr. F.
  Dept. of Urology, St. Radboud Ziekenhuis, University of Nijmegen, Nijmegen/Netherlands
EBNER, Prof. Dr. H.
  Zytologisches Labor am Zentrum für Pathologie I, Langhansstraße 10, D−6300 Gießen/FRG
EGGERS, Prof. Dr. H. J.
  Institut für Virologie der Universität Köln, Fürst-Pückler-Straße 56, D−5000 Köln 41/FRG
FINK, Dr. rer. nat. Dr. med. habil. E.
  Abteilung für Klinische Chemie und Klinische Biochemie der Chirurgischen Klinik, Nußbaumstraße 20, D−8000 München 2/FRG
FRIESEN, Dr. A.
  Urologische Abteilung des Städt. Krankenhauses, Thalkirchner Straße 48, D−8000 München 2/FRG
FURR, Dr. P. M.
  Division of Communicable Diseases, MRC Clinical Research Center, Watford Road, Harrow, Middlesex HA1 3UJ/GB
GERHARD, Ursula
  Institut für Med. Mikrobiologie, Schubertstraße 1, D−6300 Gießen/FRG
GRABER, Prof. Dr. P.
  Kantonsspital Genf, Urologische Abteilung, CH−1200 Genf/Switzerland
HAMMER, Dr. G.
  Hautklinik der Universität Düsseldorf, Abteilung für Andrologie, Moorenstraße 5, D−4000 Düsseldorf 1/FRG
HANNA, Dr. N. F.
  Division of Communicable Diseases, MRC Clinical Research Center, Watford Road, Harrow, Middlesex HA1 3UJ/GB
HOFMANN, Prof. Dr. N.
  Hautklinik der Universität Düsseldorf, Abteilung für Andrologie, Moorenstraße 5, D−4000 Düsseldorf 1/FRG
HOFSTETTER, Prof. Dr. A.
  Urologische Abteilung des Städt. Krankenhauses, Thalkirchner Straße 48, D−8000 München 2/FRG
JOHANNISSON, Prof. Dr. E.
  Kantonsspital Genf, Zentrum für Zytologie, CH−1200 Genf/Switzerland
  (Present address: Kantonsspital Basel, Frauenklinik, Zytologisches Labor, Schanzenstraße 46, CH−4031 Basel/Switzerland)
JOCHUM, Dr. rer. nat. M.
  Abteilung für Klinische Chemie und Klinische Biochemie der Chirurgischen Klinik, Nußbaumstraße 20, D−8000 München 2/FRG

KRAUSE, Prof. Dr. W.
  Medizinisches Zentrum für Hautkrankheiten, Abteilung Andrologie, Deutschhausstraße 9, D–3550 Marburg/FRG

KRAUSS, Prof. Dr. H.
  Institut für Hygiene und Infektionskrankheiten der Tiere, Frankfurter Straße 89, D–6300 Gießen/FRG

KURZ, Dr. O.
  Hautklinik der Universität Düsseldorf, Abteilung für Andrologie, Moorenstraße 5, D–4000 Düsseldorf 1/FRG

LANVERS, Dr. A.
  Institut für Virologie der Universität Köln, Fürst-Pückler-Straße 56, D–5000 Köln 41/FRG

LUDVIK, Univ.-Prof. Dr. W.
  Vorstand der Urologischen Abteilung des Krankenhauses der Barmherzigen Brüder, Garnisongasse 11/6, A–1090 Wien/Austria

MA, Dr. S. H.
  Institute for Medical Research, Santa Clara Valley Medical Center, San Jose, Calif. 95128/USA

MATTELAER, Dr. J.
  Dept. of Urology, O. L. Vrouw Hospital, B–8500 Kortrijk/Belgiun

MEARES, Dr. E. M., JR.
  Tufts University School of Medicine, New England Medical Center, Dept. of Urology, 171 Harrison Avenue, Boston, Mass. 02111/USA

MERTENS, Dr. Th.
  Institut für Virologie der Universität Köln, Fürst-Pückler-Straße 56, D–5000 Köln 41/FRG

MUNDAY, Dr. P. E.
  Division of Communicable Diseases, MRC Clinical Research Center, Watford Road, Harrow, Middlesex HA1 3UJ/GB

NOLLIN, Dr. P. DE
  Dept. of Urology, O. L. Vrouw Hospital, B–8500 Kortrijk/Belgium

PEETERS, Dr. M. P.
  St. Elisabeth-Ziekenhuis, Dept. of Medical Microbiology and Regional Public Health, Tilburg/Netherlands

POLAK-VOGELZANG, Dr. A.
  National Institute of Public Health, Bilthoven/Netherlands

RIEDEL, Dr. H. H.
  Abteilung für Frauenheilkunde im Zentrum für Operative Medizin I, Hegewischstraße 4, D–2300 Kiel 1/FRG

ROTHAUGE, Prof. Dr. C. F.
  Urologische Universitätsklinik, Klinikstraße 29, D–6300 Gießen/FRG

ROVEDA, Dipl.-Biol. M. L.
  Provinzhospital Magenta, Abteilung für Mikrobiologie, Labor, Corso Cristoforo Colombo 8, I—20144 Mailand/Italy

SCHIEFER, Prof. Dr. H. G.
  Institut für Med. Mikrobiologie, Schubertstraße 1, D—6300 Gießen/FRG

SCHIESSLER, Dr. H.
  Dermatologische Klinik und Poliklinik der Universität München, Frauenlobstraße 9—11, D—8000 München 2/FRG

SCHILL, Prof. Dr. W.-B.
  Dermatologische Klinik und Poliklinik der Universität München, Frauenlobstraße 9—11, D—8000 München 2/FRG

SCHMIDT, Prof. Dr. K. L.
  Klinik für Physikalische Medizin und Balneologie, Ludwigstraße 37—39, D—6350 Bad Nauheim/FRG

SCHMIEDT, Prof. Dr. E.
  Urologische Klinik und Poliklink der Universität München, Klinikum Großhadern, Marchioninistraße 15, D—8000 München 70/FRG

SCHÜLLER, Dr. J.
  Urologische Klinik und Poliklinik der Universität München, Klinikum Großhadern, Marchioninistraße 15, D—8000 München 70/FRG

SHEPARD, Dr. M. C.
  S. T. D. Control Laboratory, Occupational and Preventive Medicine, Regional Medical Center, Camp Lejeune, N. C. 28542/USA
  (Present address: 1008 River Street, Jacksonville, N. C. 28540/USA)

SHORTLIFFE, Dr. L. M. D.
  Urology Section, Palo Alto Veterans Administration Medical Center, Surgical Service, 3801 Miranda Avenue, Palo Alto, Calif. 94304/USA

STAMEY, Dr. T. A.
  Stanford University, School of Medicine, Dept. of Surgery, Division of Urology, Stanford, Calif. 94305/USA

STURM, Dr. W.
  Urologische Klinik und Poliklinik der Universität München, Klinikum Großhadern, Marchioninistraße 15, D—8000 München 70/FRG

SZIEGOLEIT, Dr. A.
  Institut für Med. Mikrobiologie, Schubertstraße 1, D—6300 Gießen/FRG

TAYLOR-ROBINSON, Dr. D.
  Division of Communicable Diseases, MRC Clinical Research Center, Watford Road, Harrow, Middlesex HA1 3UJ/GB

THOMAS, Dr. B. J.
  Division of Communicable Diseases, MRC Clinical Research Center, Watford Road, Harrow, Middlesex HA1 3UJ/GB
TOMMASINI-DEGNA, Dr. A.
  Provinzhospital Magenta, Institut für Pathologie, Corso Cristoforo Colombo 8, I−20144 Mailand/Italy
VEEN, Dr. J. VAN DER
  Dept. of Medical Microbiology, St. Radboud Ziekenhuis, University of Nijmegen, Nijmegen/Netherlands
WEIDNER, Priv.-Doz. Dr. W.
  Urologische Universitätsklinik, Klinikstraße 37a, D−6300 Gießen/FRG
ZANOLLO, Dr. A.
  Provinzhospital Magenta, Arbeitsgruppe Andrologie, Abteilung Urologie, Corso Cristoforo Colombo 8, I−20144 Mailand/Italy

*Division of Urology, Tufts University School of Medicine and Department of Urology,
New England Medical Center, Boston, Mass.*

Chronic Bacterial Prostatitis

E. M. MEARES JR.

Although the incidence of nonbacterial prostatitis (NBP) greatly exceeds that of chronic bacterial prostatitis (CBP), CBP is deemed a more important clinical infirmity since it is a leading cause of relapsing urinary tract infection (UTI) in men. Much of the confusion regarding the etiology and significance of prostatitis relates to nonstandard methods of diagnosis that have caused clinicians to "lump together" as "prostatitis" diseases of variable type and sequelae. Since proper therapy varies considerably according to the underlying cause of the prostatitis, careful attention must be given to diagnostic specificity.

Types of prostatitis

Nonbacterial prostatitis, the most common form of prostatitis, is characterized by excessive inflammatory cells in the prostatic expressate and symptoms that mimic those of chronic bacterial prostatitis; however, afflicted patients characteristically have no identifiable causative infectious agent and do not experience documented urinary tract infection. Bacterial prostatitis, acute and chronic, is caused by specific gram-negative or gram-positive pathogens and is characterized by the occurrence of relapsing UTI due to the pathogen that persists in the prostate. Special types of bacterial prostatitis include infections caused by the gonococcus or by the tubercle bacillus. Rarer forms include prostatic infections due to obligate anaerobic bacteria, various fungi and parasites, and nonspecific granulomatous prostatitis (eosinophilic and non-eosinophilic varieties). Currently, there is little evidence that viruses cause prostatitis. Although prostatitis due to Mycoplasmas or *Ureaplasma urealyticum* may occur infrequently, the speculation that *Chlamydia trachomatis* is a frequent or important pathogen in prostatitis remains unproved and requires further study (MARDH et al., 1978; MEARES, 1980).

Methods of diagnosis

Histologic examination of prostatic tissue is generally required to confirm a diagnosis of unusual forms of prostatitis, such as nonspecific granulomatous prostatitis; unfortunately, prostatic biopsy is not specifically diagnostic of chronic bacterial prostatitis, since conditions other than bacterial infection produce a similar appearance of tissue reaction to injury. The findings of x-ray, cystoscopy, or even rectal examination of the prostate cannot differentiate the most common types of chronic prostatitis. Moreover, both NBP and CBP are usually associated with the findings of excessive inflammatory cells (greater than 10 WBC per high power field and numerous lipid-laden macrophages); therefore, microscopic examination of the prostatic expressate is not specifically diagnostic (ANDERSON and WELLER, 1979; BLACKLOCK, 1969; MEARES, 1980).

Investigations during the past few years have clearly shown that most men with chronic bacterial prostatitis exhibit an immune response against the infective pathogen. In 1974, Gray, Billings and Blacklock used techniques of radial immunodiffusion agar plates and immunoelectrophoresis to demonstrate elevated concentrations of immunoglobulins (IgA, IgG, IgM) in the prostatic secretions of men with prostatitis (bacterial and nonbacterial) when compared to normal controls. About 80 per cent of men with chronic bacterial prostatitis due to various serogroups of *Escherichia coli* have elevated serum antibody titers against their prostatic pathogens (MEARES, 1977); furthermore, longitudinal studies show these titers tend to remain elevated or return to normal range in accordance with clinical and bacteriologic evidence of therapeutic cure or failure (MEARES, 1978). In addition, positive assays for antibody-coated bacteria have been observed in the urine of men with chronic bacterial prostatitis (THOMAS et al., 1974; JONES, 1974). More recently, a solid phase radioimmunoassay was developed to measure antigen-specific antibodies against formalinized bacterial antigens recovered from infected human prostatic secretions (SHORTLIFFE et al., 1981). These investigators have shown a distinct local antibody response in the prostatic fluid of patients with bacterial prostatitis that is independent of the serum response and that local secretory IgA is the predominant antibody in bacterial prostatitis. Although studies of the immune response offer exciting prospects for research, these techniques will not likely be available to the usual clinician who must diagnose and treat men with signs and symptoms of prostatitis.

The work of several groups of investigators has shown that bacterial prostatitis is associated with a marked secretory dysfunction of the prostate that is characterized by a marked decrease in specific gravity and diminution in concentration of most normal constituents of the secretions, including the cations (zinc, calcium, magnesium) and citric acid (MEARES, 1980). Also observed in the prostatic secretions of men with chronic bacterial prostatitis are a significant increase in alkalinity (ANDERSON and FAIR, 1976; BLACKLOCK and BEAVIS, 1974; PFAU et al., 1978), a decrease in antibacterial activity (FAIR et al., 1976), and a doubling of lactate dehydrogenase isoenzyme-5 as compared with isoenzyme-1 (GRAYHACK et al., 1980). Whereas measurement of some or all of these functional parameters may assist the clinician in establishing a diagnosis of prostatic dysfunction possibly associated with prostatic inflammation, abnormal results do not specifically differentiate one form of prostatitis from another.

The preferred method for diagnosis of bacterial prostatitis is identification of the specific infectious pathogen by means of microbial culture. Because of possible contamination by urethral organisms of nonprostatic origin, isolated culture of the prostatic expressate or ejaculate can be highly misleading. The most accurate confirmation of bacterial prostatitis is the performance of essentially simultaneous quantitative bacteriologic cultures of the urethra, bladder urine, and expressed prostatic secretions (MEARES and STAMEY, 1968).

Bacteriologic localization techniques

Collection of specimens

The voided urine and expressed prostatic secretions are partitioned into segments: the first voided 10 ml (VB1, voided bladder 1); the midstream aliquot (VB2); the prostatic secretions expressed by prostatic massage (EPS, expressed prostatic secretions); and the first voided 10 ml immediately after prostatic massage (VB3).

The patient should have a full bladder and a genuine desire to void. Skin preparation is generally unnecessary for the circumcised male. The uncircumcised male retracts his foreskin and maintains full retraction throughout collection of all specimens. The glans is cleansed with an antiseptic, such as povidone-iodine, washed with a sterile wet sponge, and dried. The first 10 ml of voided urine are collected as the patient urinates directly into a sterile tube; after about 200 ml have been emptied from the bladder, the midstream aliquot (VB2) is collected. The patient stops voiding and bends forward. As the physician systematically massages the prostate, he collects drops of prostatic fluid (EPS) directly into a wide-mouthed container. At the end of the massage, the physician exerts gentle stripping pressure on the patient's bulbar urethra to expel into the container any fluid that has pooled in the urethra during the massage. The patient immediately voids again and the first 10 ml of urine

voided (VB3) are collected in a fashion similar to that used for the VB1. Even
if insufficient EPS has been obtained for culture purposes, a cloudy VB3, when
compared to the VB1, usually means that it contains prostatic fluid.

Quantitative culture techniques

All specimens are refrigerated immediately until culture techniques are performed. When the volume is sufficient, 0.1 ml of each specimen is surface
streaked onto both blood agar and a differential medium, such as MacConkey
or eosin-methylene-blue (EMB) agar; otherwise, 0.01 ml is used by means of a
standard bacteriologic loop. After incubation for 24−48 hours, bacterial colonies are counted and multiplied by 10 (when 0.1 ml specimens are used) to
give the quantitative count of bacterial colonies per milliliter on each plate.
Standard bacteriologic methods of organism identification are then used.

Interpretation of cultures

When the bladder urine (VB2) is sterile or nearly so, pathogenic bacteria can
usually be localized to the urethra or prostate by a comparison of the bacterial
counts of the urethral and prostatic specimens. In urethral infection, the VB1
count significantly exceeds (by at least one logarithm) the counts of the EPS
and VB3 cultures. In bacterial prostatitis, the counts of the EPS and VB3
cultures should significantly exceed (by at least one logarithm) the count of the
VB1 culture.

When the bladder culture (VB2) reveals significant bacteriuria, the site of
infection cannot be accurately localized with these methods. Instead, therapy is
instituted with a drug such as nitrofurantoin, penicillin G, or ampicillin, which
will usually sterilize the urine but not the prostatic secretions. The segmented
cultures are then done 3−4 days later. Despite bactericidal levels of antimicrobial drug in the urine, the prostatic pathogens will still grow on the surface of
the agar plates of the EPS and VB3 specimens in cases of bacterial prostatitis.
Indeed, the most diagnostic pattern of bacterial prostatitis is sterile VB1 and
VB2 cultures in the presence of positive EPS and VB3 specimens. Clinical
examples of these localization cultures are shown in Table 1.

Table 1. Duplicate set of localization cultures showing reproducible pattern diagnostic of chronic bacterial prostatitis in 10 patients. In each instance the bacterial colony counts of the prostatic cultures (EPS and VB3) significantly exceed those of the urethral (VB1) and midstream (VB2) cultures. (Modified from MEARES, 1979.)

Patient	Antibiotic	Colonies per ml				Organism
		VB1	VB2	EPS	VB3	
1	Yes	0	0	1,000	0	Enterococcus
1	Yes	20	0	4,000	20	Enterococcus
2	Yes	0	0	7,000	200	P. mirabilis
2	Yes	0	0	10,000	600	P. mirabilis
3	No	1,000	300	100,000	10,000	E. coli
3	Yes	100	0	10,000	1,000	E. coli
4	Yes	0	0	7,000	10	E. coli
4	No	0	0	10,000	600	E. coli
5	Yes	250	20	5,000	400	K. pneumoniae
5	Yes	0	0	10,000	1,300	K. pneumoniae
6	No	60	0	1,000	20	E. coli
6	No	640	40	100,000	1,200	E. coli
7	Yes	0	0	600	200	E. coli
7	Yes	0	0	5,000	100	E. coli
8	Yes	0	0	600	200	E. coli
		0	0	500	30	P. mirabilis
8	Yes	0	0	400	100	E. coli
		0	0	600	50	P. mirabilis
9	Yes	50	0	100,000	5,000	K. pneumoniae
9	Yes	10	0	50,000	1,000	K. pneumoniae
10	Yes	20	0	6,000	600	E. coli
10	Yes	530	200	40,000	2,000	E. coli

Chronic bacterial prostatitis

Etiology and pathogenesis

The causative agents in bacterial prostatitis are similar in type and prevalence to those responsible for urinary tract infections. Most prostatic infections are caused by various strains of *Escherichia coli,* although infections caused by species of proteus, klebsiella, enterobacter, pseudomonas, serratia, and other less common types of gram-negative organism are sometimes found (MEARES, 1980).

Mixed infections, caused by two or more strains or classes of bacteria, occur on occasion. Although most investigators agree that the enterococcus *(Streptococcus fecalis)* is a definite prostatic pathogen that leads to relapsing urinary tract infection, the role of other gram-positive bacteria as prostatic pathogens remains controversial. Since the normal microflora of the male urethra often contains small numbers of gram-positive, nonpathogenic "skin inhabitants", such as micrococci, coagulase-negative staphylococci, streptococci, and diphtheroids, one must be cautious in considering these bacteria pathogens during interpretation of localization cultures. Some believe that gram-positive bacteria are the most common pathogens in prostatitis (DRACH, 1975). Careful longitudinal studies of patients who have only gram-positive bacteria other than enterococcus on localization cultures, however, usually show a lack of reproducibility proving bacterial prostatitis and no tendency for these organisms to cause urinary tract infections. Since these findings differ significantly from those observed in patients who have gram-negative prostatitis, many believe that chronic prostatitis due to gram-positive bacteria other than enterococcus is uncommon (MEARES, 1980; PFAU and SACKS, 1976; STAMEY, 1980).

The pathogenesis of bacterial prostatitis is often unclear. Possible routes of infection include 1. ascending urethral infection; 2. reflux of infected urine into prostatic ducts that empty into the posterior urethra; 3. invasion by rectal bacteria via direct extension or lymphatic spread; and 4. hematogenous infection.

Both gonococcal and nongonococcal urethritis develop in men by ascending infection after vaginal inoculation of the urinary meatus during sexual intercourse. Apparently, gonococcal prostatitis occurs only in men who have histories of gonococcal urethritis. A similar pathogenesis may explain some other forms of prostatitis. The male sexual partners of women who have pathogenic coliforms in their vaginal cultures often show the same bacteria in their urethral cultures (STAMEY, 1980). Usually, these men are asymptomatic and their urethral cultures often revert to normal spontaneously. However, the concomitant occurrence of identical strains of coliforms have been noted in prostatic fluid cultures in men with chronic bacterial prostatitis and in vaginal cultures from their female sexual partners (BLACKLOCK, 1974; STAMEY, 1980). Additional studies may prove that bacterial prostatitis is often a sexually transmitted disease.

Reflux of infected urine into prostatic ducts might be an important route of infection. The recent observation that many prostatic calculi contain material commonly found in urine but foreign to prostatic secretions (SUTOR and WOOLEY, 1974) suggests that urine enters the prostatic ducts, presumably by reflux, and initiates or participates in stone formation. Similarly, urethroprostatic reflux may transport bacteria from infected urine into the prostate with resultant bacterial prostatitis.

Clinical features

The clinical features of chronic bacterial prostatitis are highly variable; however, CBP is one of the most common sites of bacterial persistence leading to relapsing urinary tract infection in men. Although some men develop chronic prostatitis following an initial bout of acute bacterial prostatitis, many have no history of acute prostatitis. Some are diagnosed only because asymptomatic bacteriuria is found incidentally. Most patients experience variable irritative voiding symptoms and pain perceived at various sites (suprapubic, perineal, low back, scrotal, penile, or inner thigh areas). Some complain of postejaculatory pain and intermittent hemospermia. Unless an acute exacerbation of the chronic infection occurs, chills and fever are unusual. Although a tender, boggy prostate is often characteristic of prostatitis, these findings are not specifically diagnostic of CBP. Especially in men over the age of 35, recurrent epididymitis often denotes an underlying bacterial prostatitis.

The hallmark of chronic bacterial prostatitis is relapsing bacteriuria in which the same pathogen is found repeatedly. Despite therapy with most antimicrobic agents, the pathogen persists in prostatic fluid because most drugs diffuse poorly from plasma into prostatic ducts and acini; hence, therapeutic levels generally are not achieved in prostatic fluid. Appropriate drugs generally sterilize the urine and control many of the symptoms associated with CBP; however, discontinuation of the medication eventually leads to reinfection of the urine by the prostatic pathogen and recurrence of symptoms. Treatment failures seldom are associated with changing sensitivity of the organism to drugs.

Secretory dysfunction

Significant alterations in the composition of prostatic secretions have been observed in patients with prostatitis. In chronic bacterial prostatitis these changes are sufficiently profound to suggest an accompanying generalized secretory dysfunction of the gland (Table 2). This secretory dysfunction most likely influences the passage of drugs into prostatic fluid, especially since the secretions become more alkaline than normal in instances of CBP. Recent studies indicate that unlike the slightly acidic or slightly alkaline pH of prostatic fluid in normal men, prostatic secretions in men with chronic bacterial prostatitis are distinctly alkaline (mean of 8.0 or greater) (ANDERSON and FAIR, 1976; BLACKLOCK and BEAVIS, 1974; FAIR and CORNONNIER, 1978; FAIR et al., 1979; PFAU et al., 1978).

Human prostatic fluid contains a potent antibacterial factor (PAF) that is bactericidal to most gram-negative and gram-positive organisms. This factor

Table 2. Prostatic fluid alterations in bacterial prostatitis.
(Modified from MEARES, 1980.)

Increased
1. pH value
2. Ratio of LDH isoenzyme 5 to LDH isoenzyme 1 (LDH-5/LDH-1 = ≥ 2)
3. Immunoglobulins (IgA, IgG, IgM)
4. Complement C3 concentration
5. Transferrin concentration

Decreased
1. Specific gravity
2. Prostatic antibacterial factor (PAF)
3. Cation concentrations (zinc, magnesium, calcium)
4. Citric acid concentration
5. Spermine concentration
6. Cholesterol concentration
7. Enzyme concentrations (acid phosphatase, lysozyme)

has been identified as a compound of zinc, probably a zinc salt (FAIR et al., 1976). Since zinc concentrations are low and PAF activity is depressed or absent in men with chronic bacterial prostatitis, some believe that zinc (PAF) serves as a natural defense mechanism against ascending UTI in men. To resolve this question, one must initially determine whether men become infected because their prostatic secretions contain inadequate levels of zinc (PAF) or whether zinc (PAF) levels are depressed as a sequela of the infection. Likewise, whether men develop bacterial prostatitis because they have secretory dysfunction of the gland or whether secretory dysfunction occurs as a result if the infection remains unresolved. Although some employ the use of oral zinc preparations in the therapy of chronic prostatitis, it remains unclear whether the level of zinc in prostatic secretions is altered significantly by zinc ingestion.

Drug diffusion into prostatic secretions

Experiments performed in dogs show that most antimicrobial agents normally useful against gram-negative pathogens diffuse poorly from plasma into prostatic secretions; a notable exception is trimethoprim (TMP). Although a detailed review of pharmacokinetics in prostatitis exceeds our design, this topic has been reviewed in detail recently (MEARES, 1982). Assays of human prostatic tissue indicate that several antibacterial agents achieve potentially therapeutic levels within prostatic stroma and interstitium; however, clinical studies clearly indicate that cure of chronic bacterial prostatitis correlates best with the antimicrobial level in prostatic secretion, not tissue.

These diffusion experiments were performed in healthy dogs whose prostatic fluid was acidic. In patients with chronic bacterial prostatitis, the accompanying secretory dysfunction and increased alkalinity of the prostatic secretions compared to plasma likely alter significantly the accumulation of certain drugs in prostatic fluid. In this regard, STAMEY et al. (1973) studied the diffusion of TMP in normal dogs and observed prostatic fluid/serum ratios of 5.9 to 7.0, as compared with saliva/serum ratios of 0.7 to 0.9. The mean pH of prostatic fluid in the dogs ranged from 5.7 to 6.2, as compared with the uniformly alkaline pH of saliva (7.8 to 8.8). FAIR (1974) studied the diffusion of minocycline in dogs and noted higher levels in saliva (alkaline pH), as compared with prostatic fluid (acidic pH). Since the pH of saliva, not prostatic secretions, in dogs probably correlates best with the pH of prostatic secretions in men who have chronic bacterial prostatitis, one might speculate that drug levels obtained in canine saliva more nearly approximate those obtained in infected human prostatic fluid than do those levels noted in canine prostatic fluid.

Medical treatment

Despite theoretical concerns about the accumulation of TMP in alkaline prostatic secretions, trimethoprim-sulfamethoxazole (TMP-SMX) is the antimicrobial agent with the best documented record of success in treating CBP. Among patients who received long-term therapy (4 to 16 weeks), the cure rates have been 32% to 71%, a rate more than twice that noted with short-term therapy (MEARES, 1980). Our preference is to treat patients who have susceptible pathogens with TMP-SMX, one double-strength tablet (160 mg of TMP, 800 mg of SMX) twice daily for 12 weeks. The efficacy of using TMP alone, two tablets (100 mg of TMP each) twice daily instead of the combination is under investigation. Theoretically, when the prostatic secretions are quite alkaline, both erythromycin and minocycline may achieve therapeutic levels in the secretions against highly sensitive pathogens. Unfortunately, both drugs are characterized by a high incidence of adverse side effects and neither is suitable for long-term use. In our opinion, the preliminary studies regarding the apparent efficacy of carbenicillin indanyl sodium (Geocillin) reported by OLIVERI et al. (1979) require confirmation using longer post-therapy patient followups.

Patients not cured by medical therapy usually can be managed satisfactorily by continuous suppressive therapy with low-dose medication. Preferred regimens include TMP-SMX, one single-strength tablet daily, or nitrofurantoin,

100 mg by mouth once or twice daily. Suppressive therapy usually controls symptoms and prevents bacteriuria; however, cessation of such therapy eventually results in recurrent symptoms and bacteriuria.

Surgical treatment

Therapy by surgical means may be appropriate for patients with chronic bacterial prostatitis who cannot be managed successfully by medical therapy alone. Total prostatovesiculectomy offers the best likelihood of cure; however, the sequelae of this radical approach seldom make this procedure desirable for benign disease. Provided all foci of infected tissue and calculi are removed, transurethral prostatectomy can be curative (MEARES, 1981). Since the inflammation in chronic bacterial prostatitis occurs mainly in the peripheral portions of the gland (BLACKLOCK, 1974), complete resection is required for successful results. Our recent experience in curing several men with carefully documented chronic bacterial prostatitis not curable by medical therapy by means of "radical transurethral resection" encourage us to pursue this approach in selected patients.

Chronic calculous prostatitis

Prostatic calculi develop commonly in middle-aged and elderly men. Indeed, careful examination of surgical and autopsy specimens indicate nearly every prostate in men of this age contains prostatic calculi, most of which are tiny and invisible on x-ray films taken of the pelvis (Fox, 1963). Although prostatic stones may cause intermittent shedding of leukocytes in prostatic fluid, they generally are deemed harmless as long as they remain confined within the prostate and its ducts. However, in certain men with prostatic stones and relapsing bacteriuria, bacterial pathogens within the calculi have proved to be the source of the relapsing bacteriuria (EYKYN et al., 1974; MEARES, 1974, 1981). Similar to infected kidney stones, such prostatic calculi are impregnated to the core with bacteria that are totally protected from contact with antimicrobial agents. The successful removal of these infected calculi by surgical means is the only chance for cure.

Little is known about the formation and significance of prostatic calculi. However, urethroprostatic reflux might play an important role both in the formation of certain types of prostatic calculi and in the pathogenesis of bacterial prostatitis. Moreover, unrecognized infected calculi might play a more important role than do unfavorable pharmacokinetics in our inability to cure chronic bacterial prostatitis by antimicrobial therapy.

References

(1) ANDERSON, R. U., W. R. FAIR: Physical and chemical determinations of prostatic secretion in benign hyperplasia, prostatitis, and adenocarcinoma. Invest. Urol. *14*: 137−140 (1976).

(2) ANDERSON, R. U., C. WELLER: Prostatic secretion leukocyte studies in nonbacterial prostatitis (prostatosis). J. Urol. *121*: 292−294 (1979).

(3) BLACKLOCK, N. J.: Some observations on prostatitis. In: WILLIAMS, D. C., M. H. BRIGGS, M. STANFORD (eds.): Advances in the Study of the Prostate; pp. 37−55. William Heinemann, London 1969.

(4) BLACKLOCK, N. J.: Anatomical factors in prostatitis. Brit. J. Urol. *46*: 47−54 (1974).

(5) BLACKLOCK, N. J., J. P. BEAVIS: The response of prostatic fluid pH in inflammation. Brit. J. Urol. *46*: 537:542 (1974).

(6) DRACH, G. W.: Prostatitis: Man's hidden infection. Urol. Clin. N. Amer. *2*: 499−520 (1975).

(7) EYKYN, S., M. I. BULTITUDE, M. E. MAYO, R. W. LLOYD-DAVIES: Prostatic calculi as a source of recurrent bacteriuria in the male. Brit. J. Urol. *46*: 527−532 (1974).

(8) FAIR, W. R.: Diffusion of minocycline into prostatic secretion in dogs. Urology *3*: 339−343 (1974).

(9) FAIR, W. R., J. J. CORDONNIER: The pH of prostatic fluid: A reappraisal and therapeutic implications. J. Urol. *120*: 695−698 (1978).

(10) FAIR, W. R., J. COUCH, N. WEHNER: Prostatic antibacterial factor. Identity and significance. Urology *7*: 169−177 (1976).

(11) FAIR, W. R., D. B. CRANE, N. SHILLER, W. D. W. HESTON: A reappraisal of treatment in chronic bacterial prostatitis. J. Urol. *121*: 437−441 (1979).

(12) FOX, M.: The natural history and significance of stone formation in the prostate gland. J. Urol. *89*: 716−727 (1963).

(13) GRAY, S. P., J. BILLINGS, N. J. BLACKLOCK: Distribution of the immunoglobulins G, A and M in the prostatic fluid of patients with prostatitis. Clin. Chim. Acta *57*: 163−169 (1974).

(14) GRAYHACK, J. T., C. LEE, L. OLIVER, A. J. SCHAEFFER, E. F. WENDEL: Biochemical profiles of prostatic fluid from normal and diseased prostate glands. The Prostate *1*: 227−237 (1980).

(15) JONES, S. R.: Prostatitis as cause of antibody-coated bacteria in the urine. New Engl. J. Med. *291*: 365 (1974).

(16) MARDH, P.-A, K. T. RIPA, S. COLLEEN, J. D. TREHARNE, S. DAROUGAR: Role of Chlamydia trachomatis in non-acute prostatitis. Brit. J. Vener. Dis. *54*: 330−334 (1978).

(17) MEARES, E. M. JR.: Infection stones of the prostate gland. Laboratory diagnosis and clinical management. Urology *4*: 560−566 (1974).

(18) MEARES, E. M. JR.: Serum antibody titers in urethritis and chronic bacterial prostatitis. Urology *10*: 305−309 (1977).

(19) MEARES, E. M. JR.: Serum antibody titers in treatment with trimethoprim-sulfamethoxazole for chronic prostatitis. Urology *11*: 142−145 (1978).

(20) MEARES, E. M. JR.: Prostatitis. Ann. Rev. Med. *30*: 279−288 (1979).

(21) MEARES, E. M. JR.: Prostatitis syndromes: New perspectives about old woes. J. Urol. *123*: 141−147 (1980).

(22) MEARES, E. M. JR.: Nephrology forum: Prostatitis. Kidney International *20*: 289−298 (1981).

(23) MEARES, E. M. JR.: Prostatitis-Review of pharmacokinetics and treatment. Rev. Infect. Dis. *4*: 475−483 (1982).

(24) MEARES, E. M. JR., T. A. STAMEY: Bacteriologic localization patterns in bacterial prostatitis and urethritis. Invest. Urol. *5*: 492−518 (1968).

(25) OLIVERI, R. A., R. M. SACHS, P. G. CASTE: Clinical experience with geocillin in the treatment of bacterial prostatitis. Curr. Ther. Res. *25*: 415−421 (1979).

(26) PFAU, A., S. PERLBERG, A. SHAPIRA: The pH of the prostatic fluid in health and disease: Implications of treatment in chronic bacterial prostatitis. J. Urol. *119*: 384−387 (1978).

(27) PFAU, A., T. SACKS: Chronic bacterial prostatitis: New therapeutic aspects. Brit. J. Urol. *48*: 245−253 (1976).

(28) SHORTLIFFE, L.M.D., N. WENNER, T.A. STAMEY: The detection of a local prostatic immunologic response to bacterial prostatitis. J. Urol. *125*: 509–515 (1981).
(29) STAMEY, T.A.: Pathogenesis and treatment of urinary tract infections. Williams & Wilkins, Baltimore 1980.
(30) STAMEY, T.A., S.M.R. BUSHBY, J. BRAGONJE: The concentration of trimethoprim in prostatic fluid: Nonionic diffusion or active transport? J. Infect. Dis. (Suppl.) *128*: 686–690 (1973).
(31) SUTOR, D.J., S.E. WOLLEY: The crystalline composition of prostatic calculi. Brit. J. Urol. *46*: 533–535 (1974).
(32) THOMAS, V., A. SHELOKOV, M. FORLAND: Antibody-coated bacteria in the urine and the site of urinary-tract infection. New Engl. J. Med. *290*: 588–590 (1974).

Department of Urology, University Hospital South Manchester

Surgical Concepts in the Treatment of Chronic Bacterial Prostatitis

N. J. BLACKLOCK

Introduction

The decision regarding the surgical approach to treatment of this difficult and troublesome condition is controversial. It is essential that the condition i. e. chronic bacterial prostatitis, should be defined as specifically as is possible.

Chronic bacterial prostatitis implies the occurrence of both symptoms and signs of prostatitis over a period of several years. Fractional urine specimens and the expressed prostatic secretion will at least have shown significant evidence of the presence of inflammation i. e. leucocytosis, and cultures for micro-organisms should have been positive at least on some of the occasions. Herein there occurs the dilemma of the non-bacterial variety of this disease whose cause still eludes us although there is the evidence that *Chlamydia trachomatis* (CT) may be responsible in some (MARDH et al., 1978; SCHIEFER et al., 1983; PEETERS et al., 1983). Chronicity can only be established with the objective evidence of at least signs of an inflammatory process specifically within the prostate and the typical history of prostatic pain and voiding disturbances over a period of time coinciding with these observations and persisting in spite of the provision on at least several occasions of adequate and effective antibiotic therapy with scrupulous monitoring of pre and post treatment specimens to detect response or non-response on each occasion. In such cases there is first the possibility that anatomical factors are responsible. In this respect the natural history of the disease and the mode of infection of the gland must be considered together with various factors which are known so far to predispose to infection or to reinfection.

Surgical anatomy

All of the evidence points to an ascending route of infection in this disease which implies ingress of the infecting micro-organism into the urethra and, as a first step, the colonisation of the urethra itself. Infection probably occurs during sexual activity the mechanism of which encourages the entry of organisms into the meatus and the urethra and it is important that this basic fact be borne in mind in the context of chronic prostatitis since the treatment of the man alone without the simultaneous treatment of his sexual consort is often the reason for "chronicity" the process here being frequent reinfection from the same source (STAMEY, 1973; BLACKLOCK, 1974).

A long prepuce and − even more − a degree of phimosis with low grade balanitis ensures a higher than normal bacterial content of the fossa navicularis and again a potential source of reinfection of the urethra and perpetuation of its colonisation such as to encourage reinfection of the prostate. This factor too must therefore receive adequate consideration in the assessment of the chronic case of prostatitis.

Whilst the urethra must on many occasions be invaded by bacteria colonisation may not take place due to either the inability of the organisms to adhere to the epithelial cells or to local resistance (MARDH, COLLEEN, and HOVELIUS, 1979). In this event ascent of the organisms is unlikely. Where colonisation occurs, however, there is thereafter the possibility of further ascent to the upper urethra especially if there are the additional factors to favour this (MAYO and HINMAN, 1973; BUCK, 1975).

The urethra is held closed at two recognised sites i.e. the bladder neck and the external sphincter. The prostatic urethra between these two sphincter formations is probably also held closed by the tension of the striated sphincter of the urethra − the muscle which is mainly responsible for the observed phenomenon of "milk-back" to the neck of the bladder (Fig. 1) (CAINE and EDWARDS, 1958; BLACKLOCK, 1976). With normal urination there is relaxation of all of these sphincter complexes and the bladder empties along the lumen of the urethra. Normal micturating urethrograms frequently show a slight narrowing of the urethra due to the rigidity in the region of the external sphincter and this probably has some effect on the pressure within the prostatic urethra during urination (Fig. 2). Incomplete relaxation of this sphincter during urination will however further raise the pressure within the prostatic urethra increasing the chance of reflux into the prostatic and perhaps ejaculatory ducts (Fig. 3). Whilst failure of relaxation or sphincter dyssynergia is seen in its most gross form in neurogenic outlet obstruction persistent sphincter tension during urination is a characteristic as an irritative phenomenon in inflammatory prostatitis − accounting for the lower urine flow rate then − and also occurs with tension and anxiety when it gives rise to a similar symptom (BUCK, 1975; GEORGE and SLADE, 1979). Persistent tension even to the extent of complete sphincter closure occurs as a reflex with painful or irritative lesions in the anus and lower rectum when, again, slow urine flow rates with an interrupted stream and even urinary retention may occur. This is the basis of the so called "ano-

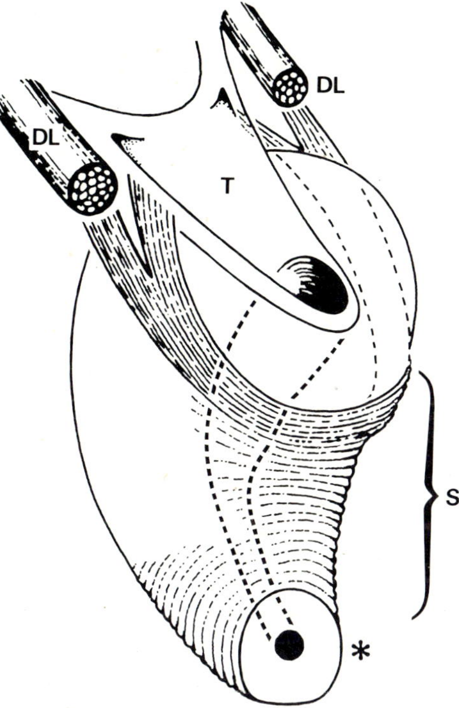

Fig. 1. Illustration of the location and extent of the striated sphincter of the urethra (S) and depicting its upper extension which encircles the urethra to find insertion in the deep trigone (T) and detrusor loop (DL). Continuous with external sphincter (★).

genital syndrome" which some regard as integral with prostatodynia (MUHRER et al., 1983; FRIESEN et al., 1983).

When urine flow is established in spite of residual sphincter tension of greater or lesser degree, turbulence in the urine flow is produced in, above and below the narrow portion of the urethra so that back-eddies of urine can lift organisms colonising the bulbous urethra higher up and into the prostatic urethra (MAYO and HINMAN, 1973). In the same circumstances due to the turbulence and raised pressure within the prostatic urethra itself it is an easy progression for microorganisms therefrom into the prostatic acini and ducts, there to set up the typical duct and acinar inflammation which characterises prostatitis (Fig. 4) (BUCK, 1975).

Just as dynamic obstruction gives rise to turbulence in flow, uplift of organisms and increase in prostatic urethral pressure so also will organic strictures or valvular formations within the urethra. Some congenital membranes may exist unnoticed by the patient who has for a long time accepted a slower urine flow

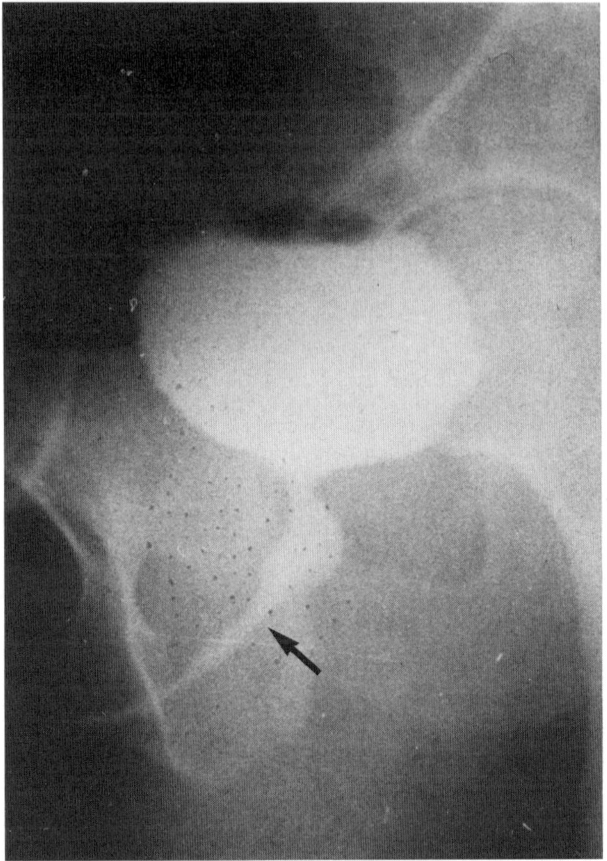

Fig. 2. Normal micturition cysto-urethrogram showing slight "pinch" effect at level of external sphincter.

than his fellows. Post-inflammatory or post-traumatic strictures, because of the acute event, will usually have presented beforehand with the complaint of a poor stream (Fig. 5).

The rarer occurrence of a urethral diverticulum causes both turbulence in urine flow and a reservoir of organisms for reinfection of the prostate.

The prostatic acinus produces a characteristic secretion containing a high concentration of zinc, acid phosphatase, citrate and a variety of enzymes. It has some resemblance in general to secretion from the salivary glands and the ionic content can lead to the formation of calculi (intrinsic) mainly formed of calcium phosphate (SUTOR and WOOLEY, 1974). These concrements may be the natural progression of some corpora amylacea, the salts forming upon a fibrinous deposit within the acinus. In this respect it is relevant that one part of the

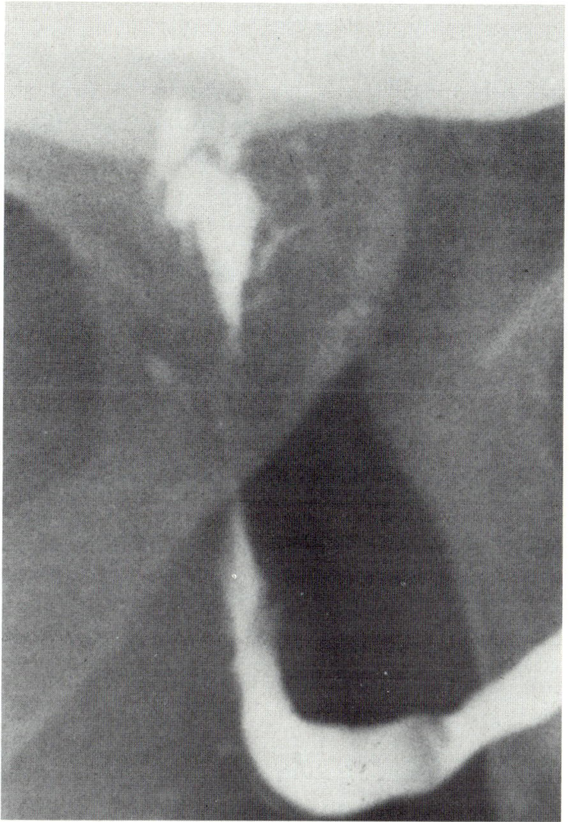

Fig. 3. Micturating cysto-urethrogram showing pronounced "pinch" effect due to incomplete relaxation of external sphincter in prostatitis leading to reflux into prostatic ducts.

prostate — the central zone — appears to be homologous with the cranial lobe of the primate prostate which is known to contain a coagulase enzyme in its secretion such that it causes a coagulum when mixed with seminal vesicular secretion (van WAGENEN, 1936; BLACKLOCK, 1976). About 50 per cent of prostatic calculi are intrinsic whilst the other half are formed from elements which can only have come from the urine i.e. calcium oxalate/phosphate and the implication from this is that there has been sufficiently frequent ingress of urine over a period of time to allow crystallisation, crystal aggregation and growth (SUTOR and WOOLEY, 1974). Prostatic calculi occur frequently and are usually asymptomatic but may account for microscopic haematuria, frank haematuria and haemospermia. When, however, infection supervenes the calculi may become reservoirs of organisms which predispose to recurrence and

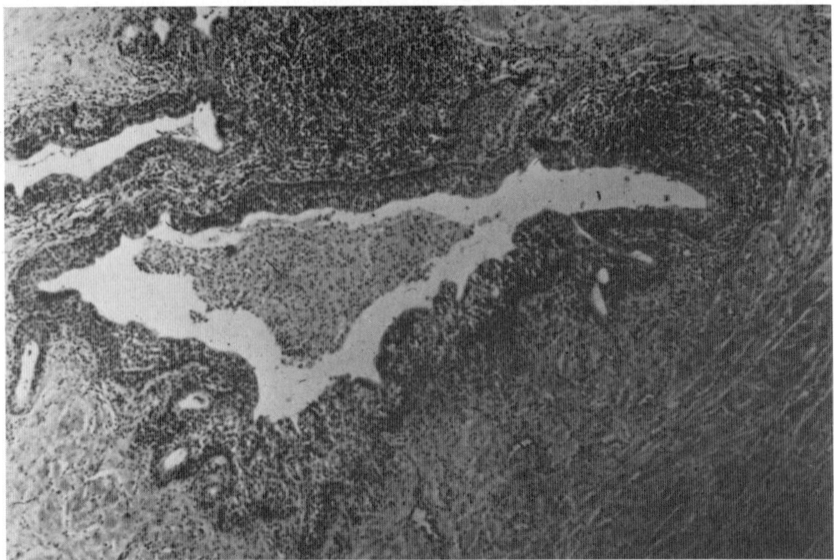

Fig. 4. Section of prostate showing inflammatory exudate in a prostatic duct and infiltration of acinar epithelium and peri-acinar tissues by leucocytes in prostatitis (H and E).

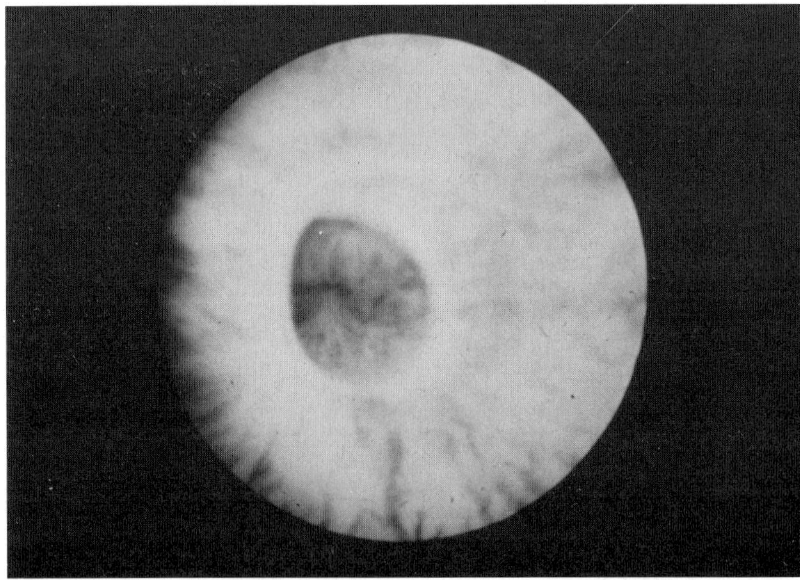

Fig. 5. Unsuspected diaphragmatic valve of bulbous urethra in case of chronic prostatitis.

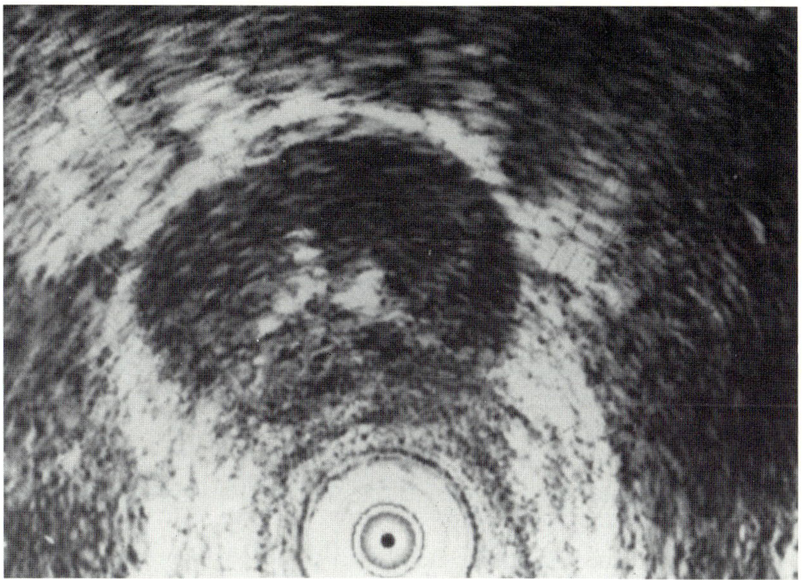

Fig. 6. Ultrasonic imaging of the prostate using a rectal probe. The hard densities within the prostate are calculi which are located alongside and behind the urethra. Mid-range echoes behind the calculi on the left side may indicate prostatitis or neoplasia. The capsule is intact. (Reproduced by courtesy of Dr. P. Brooman.)

chronicity. Rectal ultrasound scanning of the prostate and computerised tomography both demonstrate the frequency and the site of such calculi and one or both of these forms of investigation are likely to become invaluable in the assessment of cases of chronic, recurrent prostatitis (Fig. 6).

The assessment of the patient with chronic prostatitis

From the foregoing the first essential in assessment is to obtain from the patient a detailed history of the course of his disease, particular attention being paid to whether previous antibiotic treatment has been appropriate as to choice of antibiotic and adequate in duration. The adequacy of follow up will also be ascertained. It is important to obtain the evidence beyond doubt that symptoms have been due to an inflammatory form of prostatitis and the exclusion of the possibility that these are attributable to either the anogenital syndrome or urine flow and irritative phenomena due to the "anxious" bladder and its accompanying poorly relaxed external sphincter (George and Slade, 1979). Both of these basic conditions may nevertheless precipitate an active prostatitis as a result of their mechanical effects i. e. higher induced pressure in the prostatic urethra and both for the same reason may perpetuate the prostatitis as well as predisposing to it. If from the history this appears to be a main feature in the case then the overall management must include an attempt to cure the primary, predisposing condition. Any anal or rectal condition should be treated whilst continuing with the specific management of the ongoing prostatitis. Cases of anxious bladder and spastic sphincters will require psychological and even psychiatric help for cure in the longterm whilst temporary recourse may be had to alpha-adrenergic muscle relaxants (Phenoxybenzamine) or relaxants of voluntary muscle (Baclofen, Lioresal) (OSBORN et al., 1981). Antibiotic treatment of any ongoing prostatitis will continue during this time with close monitoring of the characteristics of fractional urines and the EPS.

The historical examination should also consider the sexual habits of the patient and the possibility of "chronicity" being due, in fact, to reinfection from an untreated sexual consort. If this is the case, examination, treatment and follow up of the consort is essential.

When these exclusions have been made the examination of the patient with a true refractory prostatitis will naturally include the external examination of the genitalia for phimosis and for the evidence of a previous epididymitis and funiculitis. Thereafter fractional urines and specimens of EPS should be examined as described by MEARES and STAMEY (1968) on a number of separate occasions so that a complete picture of the degree and type of infection within the prostate can be obtained.

During this time intravenous urography, endoscopy and urodynamic studies should be done together with both ascending urography and micturating cysto-urethrography. These tests may reveal the presence of the predisposing conditions already described. It is important that the endoscopy should entail complete visualisation of the urethra from the meatus upwards at the outset. The practice of passing the instrument blind and thereafter withdrawing it to obtain a view of the urethra is to be deprecated since the first passage of the instrument may destroy a soft urethral valve with very little indication what has been the cause of the condition. For the same reason urethro-cystoscopy should be carried out before ascending urethrography.

Where the facilities are available, rectal ultrasound of the prostate is invaluable since this can both locate prostatic calculi and also define the site and extent of foci of chronic inflammation (see Fig. 6). It is not possible, however, to differentiate between ultrasonic appearances of chronic prostatitis and carcinoma and the only help in this situation is the history, the findings in the EPS and the age of the patient — chronic prostatitis being more likely in the younger patient. Nevertheless there will be the occasion when prostatitis co-exists with a carcinoma in situ.

Computerised axial tomography (CT) is of some use in chronic prostatitis for its facility of showing up small areas of intraprostatic calcification. It cannot however define areas of chronic inflammatory infiltration. Both CT and rectal ultrasound can show up enlargement and inflammatory infiltration of the seminal vesicles.

Treatment

Where stenosis and balanitis co-exist with chronic prostatitis it is reasonable to recommend a circumcision to reduce the extent of colonisation of the lower urethra from this source.

Urethral folds, diaphragms and strictures should be dealt with by cold knife (Sachse urethrotomy) and thereafter the patient should be followed up by both endoscopy, urethrography and the recording of peak flow rates (PFR) (Fig. 7). Specific treatment for the chronic prostatitis should be continuous whilst normal flow rates are established and the patient thereafter will require regular follow up with assessment of PFR if nothing else to detect signs of stricture recurrence. Any indication of reduction in PFR should lead to re-examination of fractional urines and the EPS for signs of re-infection. There is the suggestion in this respect that ongoing prostatic infection may provoke recurrence (CHIARI, 1983).

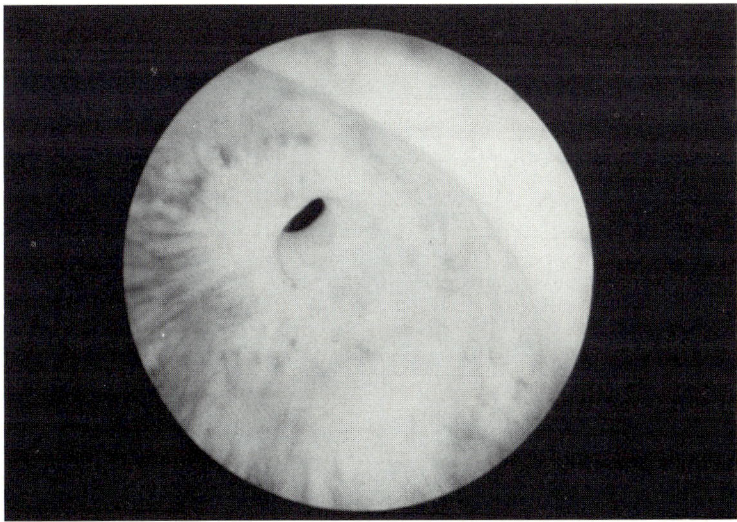

Fig. 7. Post-inflammatory stricture of the urethra in case of chronic prostatitis.

Mention has already been made of the treatment of anorectal conditions and anxiety states to overcome a tense and spastic membranous sphincter which will otherwise perpetuate infection within the prostate (OSBORN et al., 1981; READING et al., 1982).

Where prostatic calculi are demonstrated on X-Ray or ultrasound or are seen endoscopically they should be considered as niduses of infection and excised along with their loculi. There is now the possibility of operative control of this procedure by the use of real-time ultrasound in the operating theatre.

The long course of the ducts of the peripheral zone of the prostate which is that part most frequently affected by chronic prostatitis is a natural pre-disposition to chronic infection since duct obstruction by oedema or calculi can lead to stasis in a long portion of the duct and the acini which it drains (Fig. 8). Furthermore it is the ducts of the peripheral zone which lie in the lowermost part of the prostatic urethra and are therefore most accessible to organisms ascending from below and a further predisposition in their case is the peculiarity of their direction perpendicular to the line of flow down the urethra or even obliquely against this so that these are particularly vulnerable to reflux in any condition wherein the pressure within the prostatic urethra is raised and this occurs particularly during voluntary interruption of urination (Fig. 9).

These characteristics of the ducts in this part of the gland may determine the location of chronic foci of inflammation at the periphery and their focal distribution (Fig. 10). These can now be visualised ultrasonically and by this means it will be possible in the future more specifically to resect these areas and to have objective evidence of excision of the foci thereafter. During transurethral resection well established foci are usually palpable as thickenings against

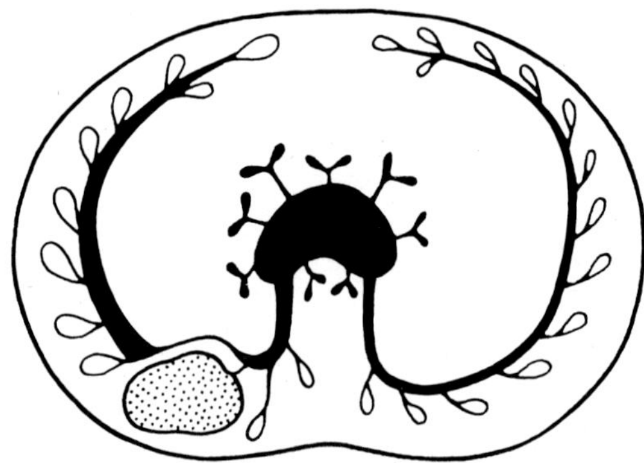

Fig. 8. Diagrammatic cross-section of the prostate showing the long course of the ducts of the peripheral zone of the prostate from their origin in the periphery of the gland to their entry into the urethra. Duct obstruction by inflammatory oedema or fibrosis may cause stasis of duct and acinar content and promote chronicity of infection.

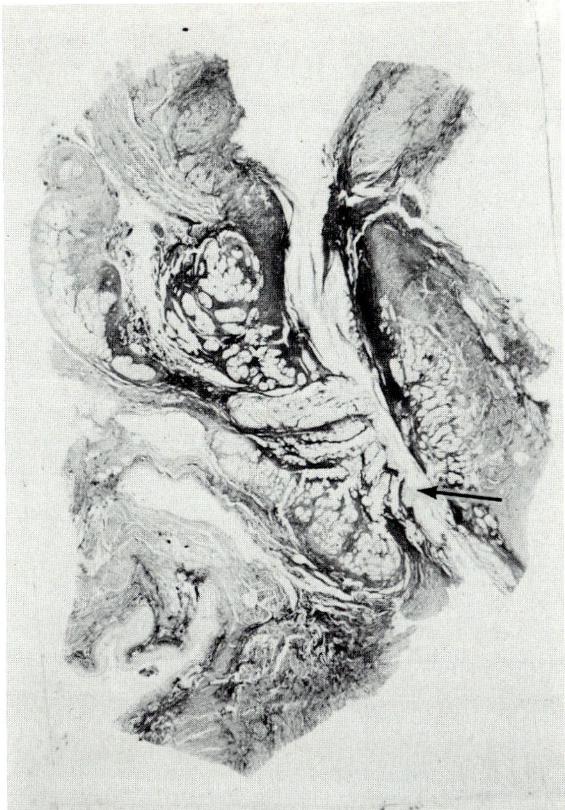

Fig. 9. Sagittal section of prostate in midline which shows direction of entry of peripheral zone ducts into urethra either perpendicular to the axis of the urethra or obliquely against the line of flow.

the sheath of the resectoscope but in view of their position in the peripheral zone the instrument has usually to be withdrawn to a level just below the verumontanum to allow access to the lesion. In order to facilitate the operative approach to a low inflammatory focus there should be control of the prostate with a finger in the rectum which pushes up on the apex of the prostate thereby placing the lesion higher and allowing access either with the loop of the resecto-scope or Collings knife without risk to the external sphincter. It is useful to gain access to the lesion first with the Collings knife since the forward direction of movement is more easy to control; defining the lesion in this way provides a marker for resection thereafter. Ultrasound techniques show the focal nature of the lesion in prostatitis and this confirms earlier experience that the policy of treatment of this condition by transurethral resection should in the first in-

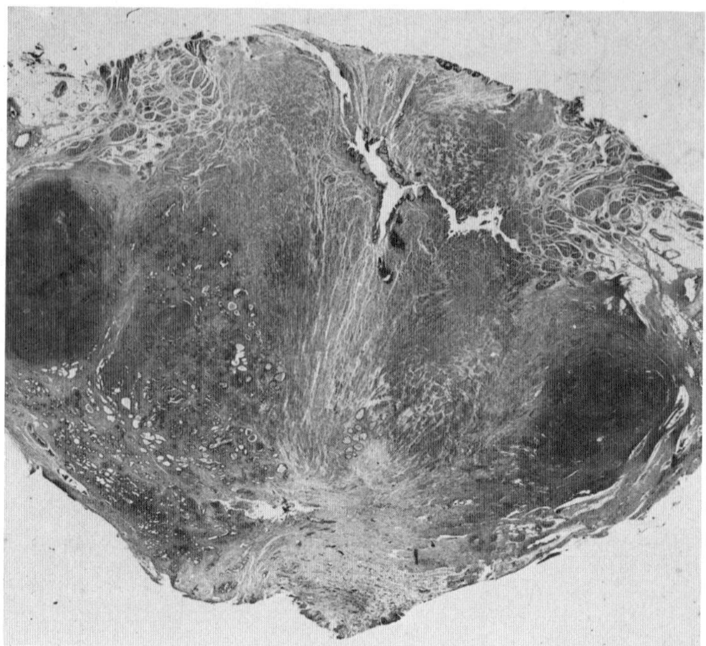

Fig. 10. Cross section of prostate showing peripheral foci of inflammation on each side (H and E).
[Reproduced by permission of *British Journal of Urology 46:* 47–54 (1974).]

stance be specifically directed at the foci of inflammation and limited to their extent. Bearing in mind the age group usually involved in this condition there is no case for indiscriminate resection of prostatic tissue including frequently normal, functional parenchyma. If there is doubt about the adequacy of any resection procedure there is advantage in a tentative philosophy, the subsequent follow up defining whether cure has been achieved.

The case against resection of the bladder neck

There is no case to support transurethral resection of the bladder neck in chronic prostatitis. The apparent indication in those cases in whom this has been done has been the poor urine flow rates both complained of and observed by the uroflowmeter. Flow rate however is determined in this instance not usually by any confinement at the bladder neck but by the incomplete relaxation of the external sphincter for which a combination of medicinal, psychological and psychiatric treatment may be needed together with reassurance on the part of the physician (OSBORN et al., 1981; READING et al., 1982).

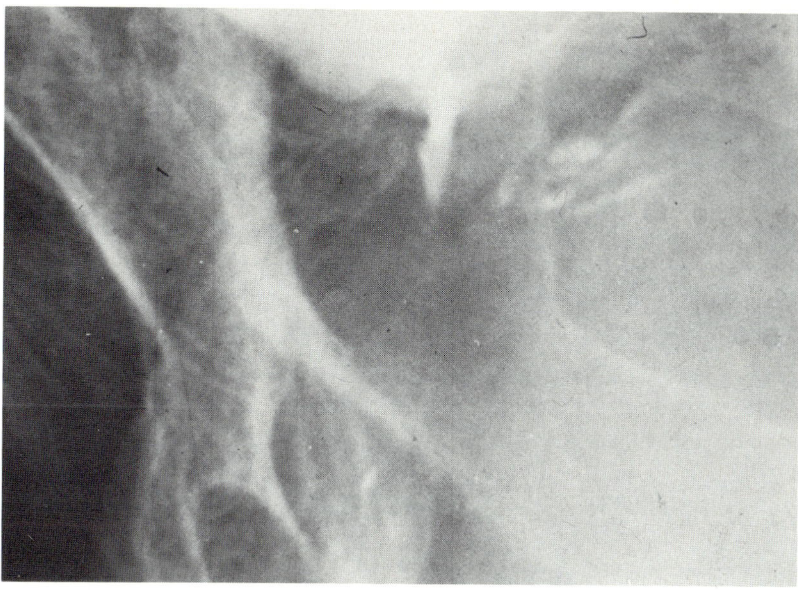

Fig. 11. Resting cystogram in case of prostatitis following bladder neck resection. Contrast medium shows communication between bladder and prostatic urethra and there is reflux into prostatic ducts on the left side.

Experience has shown that the poor urine flow rates in chronic prostatitis persist unchanged following resection of the bladder neck indicating the cause to lie at a lower level (OSBORN et al., 1981).

Quite apart from failing to relieve symptoms and result in a better urine flow, however, the resection of the bladder neck adds a further predisposition to the persistence or recurrence of infection within the prostate. With an intact bladder neck the prostatic urethra is protected by it from the surges and variations of intravesical pressure except when there is momentary relaxation of this sphincter with a very full bladder. Destruction of the bladder neck mechanism either by resection or by effective sphincterotomy means that there is continuous communication between the bladder and prostatic urethra, the prostatic urethra containing urine which is subject to all of the fluctuations of the bladder pressure which can only mean the greater frequency or even constancy of urinary reflux into the ducts of the prostate (Fig. 11). In the circumstances of an already established chronic prostatitis this can only mean a perpetuation of the condition and the ultimate destruction of the functioning parenchyma of the gland with the requirements of an extensive resection procedure and virtual ablation of the gland in due course.

For this reason the specificity of resection of focal inflammation within the prostate should try to avoid interfering with the integrity of the bladder neck mechanism itself.

Conclusion

The better and earlier recognition of the occurrence of bacterial prostatitis and improved concepts of the adequacy and effectiveness of treatment both of bacterial and non-bacterial varieties when properly applied should diminish the number of cases who end up with chronic infection of the parenchyma of the gland. The advantage of imaging techniques which can now define the exact location and extent of chronic infection are grounds for optimism for more effective surgical treatment when this becomes necessary.

There is no case for recourse to surgical management until the preliminaries of case identification and full assessment have been completely satisfied.

Bladder neck resection should never be carried out in the presence of an established prostatitis.

References

(1) BLACKLOCK, N. J.: The Anatomy of the Prostate. In: CHISHOLM G. D., D. I. WILLIAMS (eds.): Scientific Foundations of Urology; pp. 113–125. W. Heinemann, London 1976.

(2) BUCK, A. C.: Disorders of Micturition in Bacterial Prostatitis. In: Proceedings of the Royal Society of Medicine 68: 508–511 (1975).

(3) CAINE, M., D. EDWARDS: The Peripheral Control of Micturition; a Cineradiographic Study. Brit. J. Urol.: 30: 34–42 (1958).

(4) CHIARI, R.: Harnröhrenenge und Prostatitis. (Urethral Stricture and Prostatitis.) In: BRUNNER, H., W. KRAUSE, G. F. ROTHAUGE, W. WEIDNER (Hrsg.): Chronische Prostatitis. Internationale Arbeitstagung, Bad Nauheim 1981. Schattauer, Stuttgart–New York 1983.

(5) FRIESEN, A., W. FRANK. W. STREIFINGER, A. HOFSTETTER, A. REICHELT: Adnexitis und Anogenitalsyndrom. (Adnexitis and Anogenital Syndrome.) In: BRUNNER, H., W. KRAUSE, G. F. ROTHAUGE, W. WEIDNER (Hrsg.): Chronische Prostatitis. Internationale Arbeitstagung, Bad Nauheim 1981. Schattauer, Stuttgart–New York 1983.

(6) GEORGE, N. J. R., N. SLADE: Hesitancy and Poor Stream in Neurologically Normal Younger Men without Outflow Tract Obstruction. Brit. J. Urol.: 51: 506–510 (1979).

(7) MARDH, P. A., S. COLLEEN, B. HOVELIUS: Attachment of Bacteria to Exfoliated Cells from the Urogenital Tract. Invest. Urol. 16: 322–326 (1979).

(8) MARDH, P. A., K. T. RIPA, S. COLLEEN, J. D. TREHARNE, S. DAROUGAR: Role of Chlamydia trachomatis in Non-Acute Prostatitis. Brit. J. Ven. Dis. 54: 330–334 (1978).

(9) MAYO, M. E., F. HINMAN: Role of Midurethral High Pressure Zone in Spontaneous Bacterial Ascent. J. Urol.: 109: 268–272 (1973).

(10) MEARES, E. M., T. A. STAMEY: Bacteriologic Localisation Patterns in Bacterial Prostatitis and Urethritis. Invest. Urol. 5: 492–518 (1968).

(11) Muhrer, K. H., W. Weidner, D. Filler, T. Kaths: Proktologische Befunde beim vegetativen Urogenitalsyndrom (Proctological Findings in Vegetative Urogenital Syndrome). In: Brunner, H., W. Krause, G. F. Rothauge, W. Weidner (Hrsg.): Chronische Prostatitis. Internationale Arbeitstagung, Bad Nauheim 1981. Schattauer, Stuttgart–New York 1983.

(12) Osborn, D. E., N. J. R. George, P. N. Rao, R. J. Barnard, N. J. Blacklock: Prostatodynia: Physiological Characteristics and their Rational Mangement with Muscle Relaxants. Brit. J. Urol. *53*: 621–623 (1981).

(13) Peeters, M., A. Polack-Vogelzang, F. Debruyne, J. van der Veen: Abakterielle Prostatitis: Mikrobiologische Daten (Abacterial Prostatitis, Microbiological Data). In: Brunner, H., W. Krause, G. F. Rothauge, W. Weidner (Hrsg.): Chronische Prostatitis. Internationale Arbeitstagung, Bad Nauheim 1981. Schattauer, Stuttgart–New York 1983.

(14) Reading, C., D. Osborn, N. J. R. George, C. Marklow, N. J. Blacklock: Prostatodynia: A preliminary psychophysiological investigation (in press).

(15) Schiefer, H.-G., W. Weidner, W. Krause, U. Gerhardt, H. Krauss: Prostatitis nach nicht-gonorrhoischer Urethritis – Eine prospektive Untersuchung. Prostatitis: A Prospective Study of Patients with Non-Gonococcal Urethritis. In: Brunner, H., W. Krause, G. F. Rothauge, W. Weidner (Hrsg.): Chronische Prostatitis. Internationale Arbeitstagung, Bad Nauheim 1981. Schattauer, Stuttgart–New York 1983.

(16) Stamey, T. A.: The Role of Introital Enterobacteria in Recurrent Urinary Infection. J. Urol.: *109*: 467–472 (1973).

(17) Sutor, D. J., S. E. Wooley: The Crystalline Composition of Prostatic Calculi. Brit. J. Urol.: *46*: 533–535 (1974).

(18) Wagenen, G. van: The Coagulating Function of the Cranial Lobe of the Prostate Gland in the Monkey. Anat. Rec. *86*: 411–421 (1936).

Department of Urology, O. L. Vrouw Hospital, Kortrijk

Treatment of Chronic Bacterial Prostatitis by Local Injection of Antibiotics into Prostate

L. BAERT, J. MATTELAER, P. DE NOLLIN

When the patient and when we ourselves have sufficient diagnostic courage, we may be able to select from the group of "prostatitis" patients a small number of cases of bacterial prostatitis, and from them, a hard-core subgroup of patients who can be designated as chronic bacterial prostatitis. In practice, the diagnosis is not easy (1, 2, 3). The urologist and the bacteriologist have to take their samples with extreme care and must interpret them rigorously. In our method, VB2 is replaced by suprapubic puncture (SPP) (4). The interval between the last micturition and the PE is thus at least 3 to 4 hours. If the SPP (urine) and the PE have the same bacterial growth, the patient is treated with nitrofurantoin or ampicillin until a negative urine culture is obtained. If the prostatic fluid remains purulent with the same bacterial growth, a diagnosis of bacterial prostatitis is accepted.

The adjunctive diagnostic tests are the prostatic fluid − pH and the ACB[1] test with culture of the ejaculate (5). In our group of patients, the diagnosis of chronic bacterial prostatitis was based on the following findings:
1. persistent purulent prostatic fluid,
2. bacterial growth in the prostatic fluid with alcaline pH,
3. preferably bacterial growth and a positive ACB test of the ejaculate,
4. persistence of these 3 conditions after 3 weeks of oral trimethoprim-sulfamethoxazole (Co-trimoxazole) complemented by oral thiamphenicol or doxycycline for 10 days.

In our experience, a gram-negative coliform organism is practically the most frequent causative organism in chronic bacterial prostatitis. Based on theoretical characteristics as well as on experimental and clinical findings, a variety of antibacterial agents have been presented during the last decade as drugs which may be effective in curing infections of the prostate gland. Of these agents the combination of trimethoprim-sulfamethoxazole is currently the drug of first-choice in treatment of patients with chronic bacterial prostatitis. However, clinical experience revealed that using trimethoprim-sulfamethoxazole or other

---

[1] ACB: Antibody Coated Bacteria.

antimicrobial agents, a permanent cure of prostatic infection was achieved only partially.

For those patients who did not respond to antimicrobial therapy, the alternative for cure of this disease was total or transurethral prostatectomy. Transurethral resection of prostate can be curative but only if all infected foci are removed successfully.

In 1975 we reintroduced the use of intraprostatic antibiotic injections in the treatment of chronic recurrent bacterial prostatitis (6, 7, 8). The primary purpose of this report is to publish our experiences with localized antibiotic treatment of chronic bacterial prostatitis by direct injection into the prostate. We will first discuss the method we use; second, we will answer the question of whether or not these antibiotics actually reach the prostate; third, we will deal with the possible damaging effects of this therapy; and fourth, we will try to evaluate the therapeutic value of this treatment.

1. The method is simple. The antibiotic is injected by means of a long, fine needle into the caudal prostate under rectal control. The injections are generally done under local anesthesia. The antibiotics are diluted in xylocain

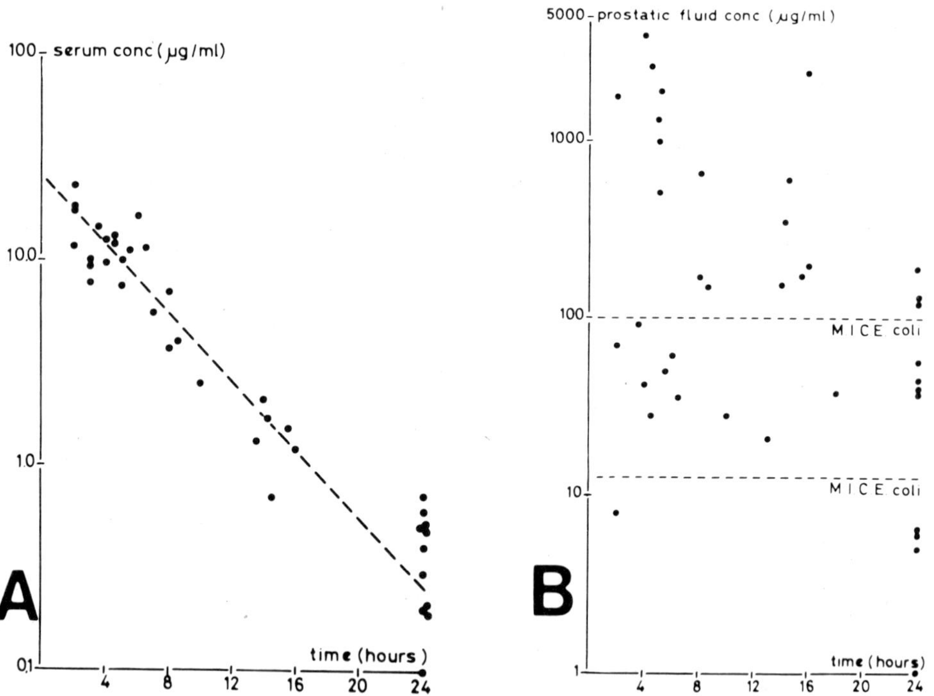

Fig. 1. Serum (A) and prostatic fluid (B) concentrations of thiamphenicol on logarithmic scale versus time after injection of 2 g thiamphenicol glycinate into prostate.

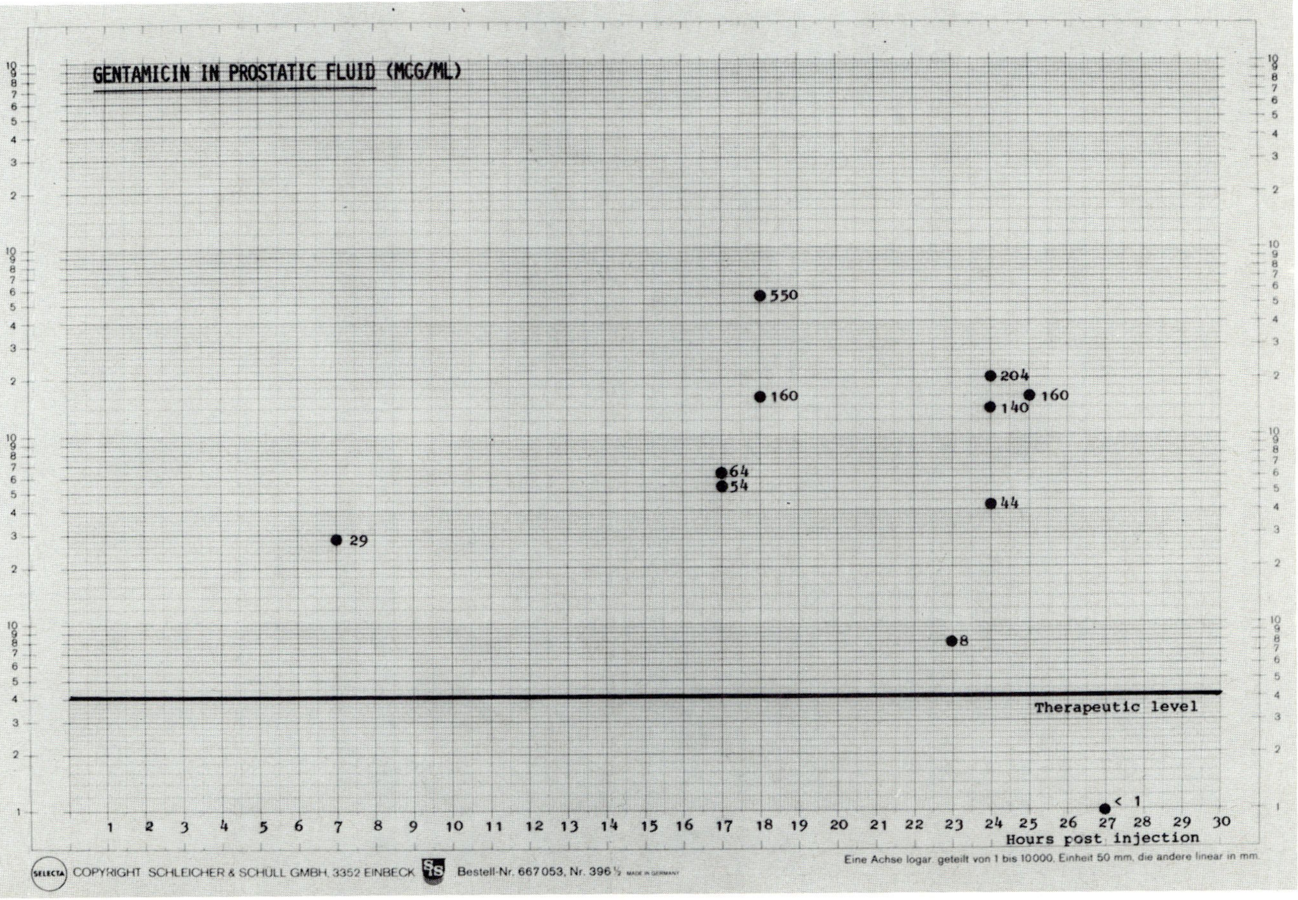

Fig. 2. Gentamicin in prostatic fluid (µg/ml).

and 0.9% NaCl-solution to a total volume of 20 ml. During the injection, the needle is frequently relocated in order to obtain the best possible distribution, a kind of floating of the prostate lobes. The position of the needle is kept under constant rectal control. We injected amikacin (3×500 mg), cefazolin (3 g), gentamicin (240 mg) and thiamphenicol glycinate (2.0 g).

2. Do these antibiotics actually reach the prostatic fluid after injection? Thiamphenicol concentration in serum and prostatic fluid at various times after injections of 2 g thiamphenicol glycinate directly into the prostate are shown in Fig. 1 (9). The thiamphenicol concentration is plotted on a logarithmic scale with the serum and prostatic fluid along the ordinate and the time after injection along the abcissa. The serum half-life of thiamphenicol is 3.6 hours. Therefore, during the 24-hour observation period, the serum concentration decreases from 25 to 0.3 micrograms per millimeter. You can see that there is no correlation between the antibiotic concentration in the prostatic fluid and the time after injection. Very high levels are found without correlation with the time after the injection for this observation period,

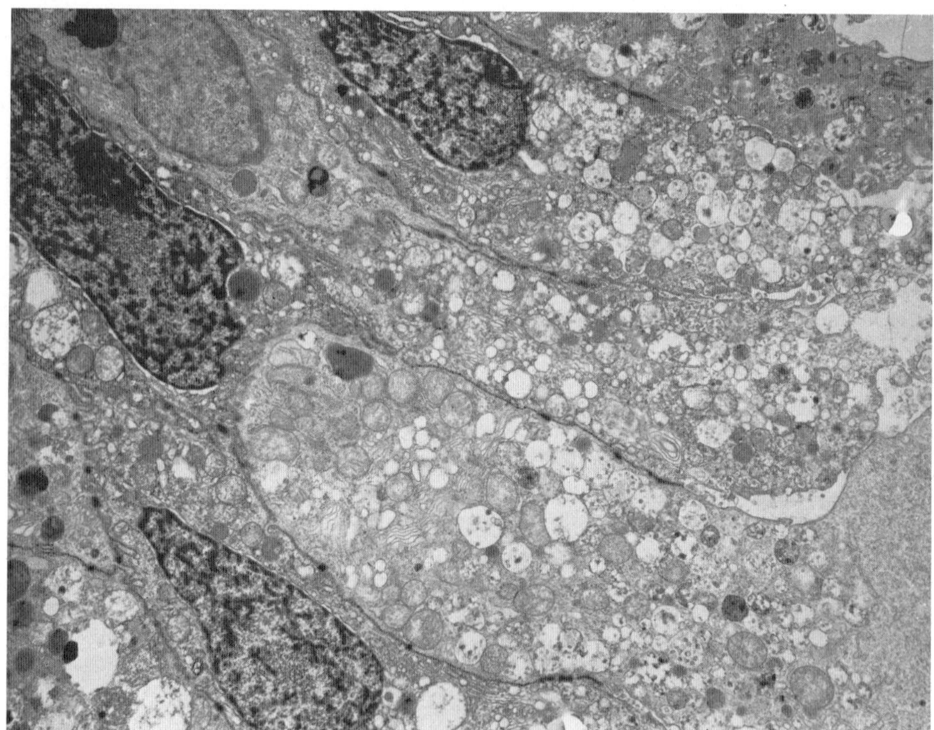

Fig. 3. Prostatic epithelia showing amino sugar acumulation in lysosomes (dense circular structures).

which was as much as 24 hours. Here, the levels vary between 1 and 4000 µg per ml. Minimum inhibitory concentration of thiamphenicol for *E. coli* is between 12.5 and 100 micrograms per ml. This zone has been outlined in Fig. 1 (B). Irrespective of the time of administration, it can be concluded that effective thiamphenicol levels, for most strains of *E. coli* are reached in the prostatic fluid of most patients.

Fig. 2 gives the gentamicin level in the prostatic fluid after local injection of 240 mg of gentamicin in the prostate. Prostatic fluid levels were determined between 8 and 27 hours after injection. The gentamicin concentration in the prostatic fluid on logarithmic scale indicates that the result is strongly dependent on the injection-technique. Only 1 out of the 11 values obtained is below the therapeutic range.

3. What are the possible damaging effects of this therapy? The pain and discomfort experienced by the patients during direct injection into the prostate are minimal and comparable to that observed after intramuscular injection. Intraprostatic injections during acute exacerbations of infection are contra-

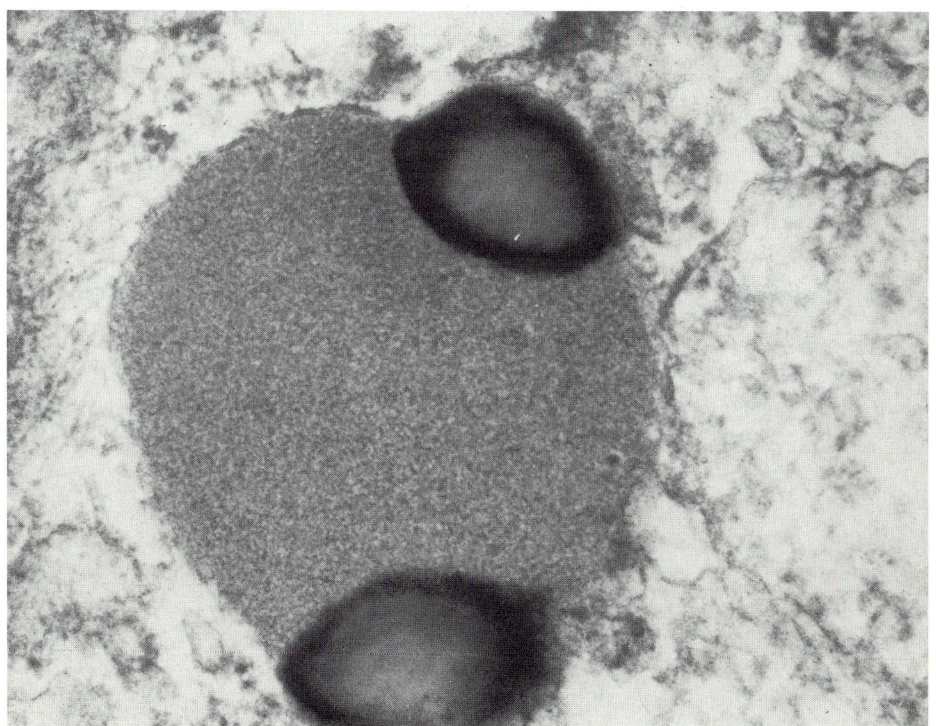

Fig. 4. Details from Fig. 3.

                   L. Baert et al.

indicated because of the danger of general dissimination of infection and septicemia. Hematuria and hemospermia during some weeks are practically always present after the injection. Retention was exceptionally observed in cases with superimposed prostatic hypertrophy. Local necrosis, a theoretical possibility, was not found after several histological and electronic microscopic studies. Fig. 3 shows a secretory acinar cell with lysosome where dense circular structures were identified. These dense structures are representative of aminosugar accumulation in lysosomes; detail are shown in Fig. 4.

Figs. 3 and 4 were obtained in a patient treated because of bacterial prostatitis, and biopsy was performed 5 months after 240 mg gentamicin injection into prostate.

4. What is the therapeutic value of this treatment method? In fact, practically all cases of chronic bacterial prostatitis can be cured by this method if the

Table 1. 44-year-old patient with recurrent urinary infections (details see text).

Dates of Infection	VB1	SPP	EPS	VB3	pHPS	ACB-Ejaculate	L.A.
1976							**1976**
9.11.		E. coli	E. coli		8.7	E. coli pos.	25.11. Gentamicin
							3× 80 mg + V
7.12.		0	0			0 negative	
1977							**1977**
14.2.		0	0			0 negative	
31.3.		E. coli	?	E. coli		E. coli pos.	
7.4.		–	E. coli			– –	7. 4. Gentamicin
7.5.		0	?				7. 5. Cefazoline 3× 1 g
16.6.		E. coli	?	E. coli	8.5		21. 6. Cefazoline
25.7.		E. coli	E. coli				25. 7. Cefazoline
							24.10. Thiamphenicol
							4× 500 mg
1978							**1978**
4.1.		E. coli	?		–	– –	
							27.2. Thiamphenicol
25.5.		E. coli	E. coli		–	– –	
							26.9. Gentamicin
5.12.		–	–		–	0 negative	
1979							**1979**
18.1.		0	0		8.1	0 negative	
4.4.		0	0		7.5	0 negative	
10.5.		0	0		–	– –	
14.6.		0	0		–	0 negative	
22.7.		0	0		–	– –	

injections are repeated regularly. Three cases have been selected from the hard-core group for illustration.

Case 1: A 44-year-old patient with recurrent urinary tract infections was treated for 3 years with various antibiotics (Table 1). After careful diagnosis, he received the first local injection of antibiotics into prostate in november 1976. The first injection produced negative cultures for 3 months, after which the cultures again showed growth of pathogenic bacteria. This was a relapse rather than a reinfection, in my opinion, and a 3 month follow-up seems to be too short a time to conclude that the patient was cured. Eight injections were administered over a period of about 2 years. A bacteriological cure was obtained that has been confirmed by a prolonged follow-up period. No oral or parenteral antibiotics were administered in the meantime.

A vesiculography (Fig. 5) was conducted at the time of this patient's first local injection and showed atrophic abortive structures and progressively shriveled semen vesicles. This is very often found in the chronic bacterial prostatitis group. Indeed, in these cases we can observe infection of the entire genito-urinary sinus involving the prostate gland and the semen vesicles. After vesiculography, the system is rinsed with isobetadin, and a sclerotizing agent is injected through the spermatic ducts.

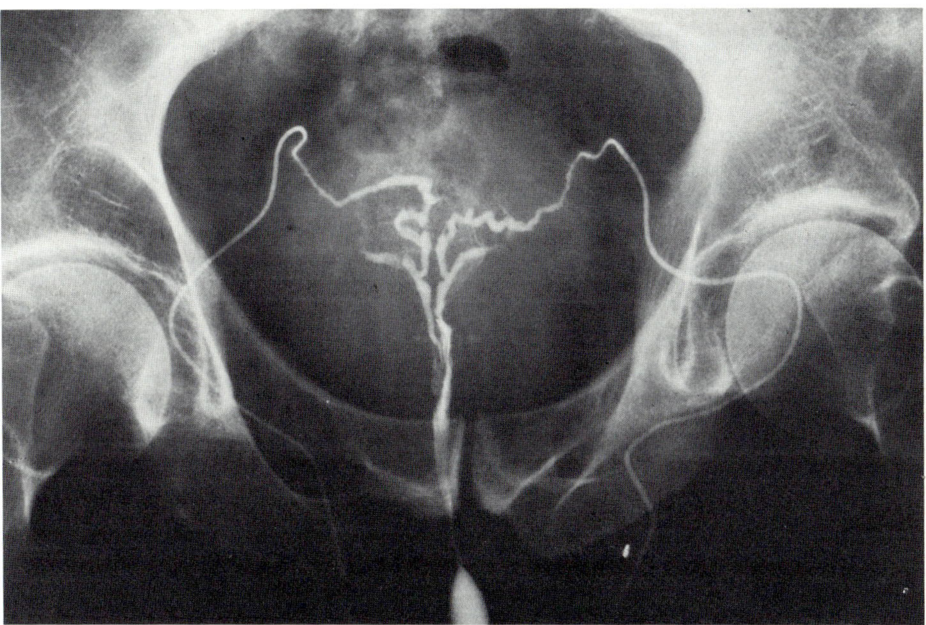

Fig. 5. Vesiculography showing atrophic abortive structures and shriveled seminal vesicles.

Table 2. 61-year-old patient with recurrent urinary infections (details see text).

Dates of Infection	VB1	SPP	EPS	VB3	pHPS	ACB-Ejaculate	L.A.
1977 8.11. 22.12.	 –	 E. coli –	 E. coli E. coli	 – –	 8.4 –	 – –	**1977** 14.11. Gentamicin 3× 80 mg
1978 14.3. 25.5. 22.9.		 0 0 0	 E. coli E. coli 0				**1978** 18.1. Thiamphenicol 4× 500 mg 25.5. Gentamicin
1979							**1979**
1980 20.12.				T⁰ + systemic signs			**1980** Reinfection(?)
1981 7.1. 3.2. 6.7. 4.8.		 E. coli E. coli 0 0	 E. coli ? 0 0		 8 – 7.4 –		**1981** 7.1. Gentamicin 18.3. Gentamicin + V

Case 2: For a 61-year-old patient, 3 injections were needed in order to obtain the first negative culture at a control examination 4 months after injection (Table 2). The patient was then free of symptoms for 2 years, at which time a new inflammatory response occurred with systemic symptomatology: fever, shivering, etc. Was this a reinfection or a relapse? Negative cultures were again obtained after 2 injections. This case illustrates how difficult it is to distinguish between a relapse and a reinfection. Incidentally, the vesiculography of this patient showed a pattern that is entirely comparable with the first case, namely, atrophic structures.

Case 3: A 34-year-old patient presented bilateral orchiepididymitis and was treated unsuccessfully for 3 months with trimethoprim-sulfamethoxazole (Table 3). Five injections were needed to eradicate the causative organism. Bacteriological cure was finally obtained with gentamicin after the failure of thiamphenicol and cefacidal.

Table 3. 34-year-old patient with bilateral orchiepididymitis (details see text).

Dates of Infection	VB1	SPP	PE	VB3	pHPS	ACB-Ejaculate	L.A.
1977 2.5.		E. coli	?				**1977**
30.6.		E. coli	E. coli		8.3		
							7. 7. Cefazoline 3× 1 g
							13. 8. Cefazoline
11.10.		E. coli	?			E. coli pos.	14.10. Thiamphenicol
							4× 500 mg
19.12.		E. coli	E. coli				
1978 25.5.		E. coli	?			E. coli pos.	**1978** 30.5. Gentamicin
							3× 80 mg
							6.7. Gentamicin
							3× 80 mg
8.8.		negative	negative			−	
1979 23.3.		negative	negative		7.2	negative	**1979**
5.5.		negative	negative				
1980 3.2.		negative	negative		7.2	negative	**1980**

Conclusion

Results after local injection of antibiotics into prostate demonstrated that this method deserves its place in our therapeutic repertoire. The advantage of this treatment is that it places a very high concentration of the antibiotic at the focus of the infection without any risk of metabolic inactivation.

References

(1) MEARES, E. M. jr., T. A. STAMEY: The diagnosis and management of bacterial prostatitis. Brit. J. Urol. *44*: 175 (1972).
(2) MEARES, E. M. Jr.: Prostatitis, a review. Urol. Clin. North Am. *2*: 3 (1975).
(3) MEARES, E. M.: Prostatitis. Kidney Intern. *20*: 289 (1981).
(4) BAERT, L.: Urine analysis estimation of residue and cystography using the suprapubic approach. Ann. Urol. *7*: 83 (1973).
(5) BLACKLOCK, N. J., J. P. BEAVIS: The response of prostatic fluid pH in inflammation. Brit. J. Urol. *46*: 537 (1974).

(6) Baert, L., H. Soep, J. Pyck: Chronische bacteriële Prostatitis. Tschr. geneesk. *16: 794 (1975).*

(7) Baert, L.: Chronic bacterial prostatitis. Ann. Urol. *10*: 39 (1976).

(8) Baert, L.: Bacterial prostatitis treated by local antibiotics, letter to the editor. Urol. *8*: 644 (1976).

(9) Baert, L., T. A. Plomp, R. A. Maes: Treatment of recurrent chronic bacterial prostatitis by local injection of thiamphenicol into prostate. Urol. *15*: 3 (1980).

S.T.D. Control Laboratory, Occupational and Preventive Medicine,
Naval Regional Medical Center, Camp Lejeune, N.C.

Role of Ureaplasma urealyticum in Male Lower Genital Tract Infections

M. C. Shepard

Ureaplasma urealyticum was first isolated nearly three decades ago by Shepard (14) from men suffering from non-gonococcal urethritis (NGU), and a possible *causative* role for *U. urealyticum* in this disease was first suggested by the same author (15, 16). Its role as an etiologic agent of NGU in the male, however, has been a subject of continued controversy.

During the 14 years between 1962 and 1976, the results of primary isolation studies of ureaplasmas from men with NGU served only to perpetuate confusion concerning the role of this organism in NGU. In 31 different controlled studies during this period, as summarized by Taylor-Robinson and McCormack (23), 17 studies *supported* an associative role of ureaplasmas in NGU, whereas 14 studies *failed* to find any evidence in support of an etiological role in NGU. Two factors which contributed to differences between the results of one study and another were the selection of inappropriate control subjects, and technical factors, such as inappropriate culture media and/or lack of expertise in identification of ureaplasmas in primary cultures. Almost none of the studies during this period included a search for *Chlamydia trachomatis*. Such studies, therefore, in the light of present knowledge concerning the important role of chlamydia in approximately 40% of NGU patients (24), are difficult to interpret. In three separate studies reported by Bowie et al. (1, 4, 5), and in a similar study reported by Wong et al. (29), ureaplasmas were isolated more frequently and in larger numbers (5) from chlamydia-negative men with NGU, than from chlamydia-positive men with NGU. In the study by Wong et al. (29), a significant association of 76% was found for ureaplasmas in men with chlamydia-negative NGU, whereas among the controls, only 31% of men without urethritis yielded ureaplasmas. Taylor-Robinson et al. (26), however, failed to observe a higher recovery rate of ureaplasmas from chlamydia-negative men in England.

One of the arguments against ureaplasmas as a cause of NGU in the male has been the rather frequent occurrence of the organism in sexually active *normal* individuals. Data originally from McCormack et al. (12) have sometimes been used to suggest that colonization by genital ureaplasmas among healthy, sexually active university men is a function of the *number* of different female sexual partners experienced — the isolation rate increasing from 19% to 45% with increasing number of different partners. None of these men developed NGU during the study. However, among the 178 men in this study, the overall *Ureaplasma* isolation rate was only 29%. This figure is similar to a *carrier rate* of 30% among 580 healthy U.S. Marine controls *without* urethritis at Camp Lejeune, N. C. This study included both men denying sexual intercourse and those admitting sexual intercourse. In contrast, among 219 men *with NGU*, 151 (69%) were positive for ureaplasmas in this controlled study by Shepard (17).

The question has been asked: Can a causal role for ureaplasmas in NGU be reconciled with the frequency with which ureaplasmas are recovered from sexually active men in whom urethritis is absent? This question was addressed 11 years ago by Shepard (16) who stated that many of the ureaplasmas isolated from healthy men without urethritis were probably commensal, non-pathogenic strains, or potentially pathogenic strains under certain (but unknown) conditions. It is therefore suggested to give consideration to the concept of asymptomatic *carriers* of genital ureaplasmas among sexually active men without urethritis, whose strains may prove to be dissimilar from pathogenic ureaplasma strains associated specifically with genital tract infections in both the male and the female. It may be recalled that carrier rates of *Neisseria meningitidis,* for example, among servicemen without evidence of meningococcal disease, were reported as high as 50—65%, at a U.S. Naval Training Center (13).

The existence in humans of both virulent and avirulent (carrier) ureaplasmas is suggested by the findings of Howard et al. (10), who reported that both virulent and avirulent strains of *bovine* ureaplasmas exist. Pathogenicity of bovine ureaplasmas was shown *not* to be characteristic of any particular serotype. It is clearly difficult to extrapolate the results achieved in animals directly to humans, but neither can such results be ignored. Fodor (8) in a limited study, reported that freshly-isolated human genital ureaplasmas differed in virulence, employing a mouse intra-renal inoculation method. Only freshly-isolated ureaplasma strains were suitable, because subcultured strains lost "mouse virulence" within a few passages. There is now a pressing need for studies comparing the biological properties of genital ureaplasmas from normal, healthy *carriers* with ureaplasmas isolated from men with urethritis and prostatitis. Biotyping studies of these two groups of ureaplasmas may eventually identify specific markers for virulence and recognition of pathogenic strains among the human ureaplasmas. In addition to the types of studies discussed above, the following types of studies strongly support a causal role for *U. urealyticum* in male genital tract disease.

Urinary mucous threads

The presence of mucous threads in first-glass urine specimens from male NGU patients is one of the characteristic features of the disease, and is an important clinical sign in the diagnosis of NGU. Following completion of therapy, the disappearance of mucous threads from the urine is important in assessing satisfactory response to treatment and cure. SHEPARD (18) observed a frequent, close association of ureaplasmas with urinary mucous threads from men with NGU, employing a special differential agar (19, 20). Such mucous threads also contain very large numbers of PMN leukocytes. Urinary mucous from normal, healthy *Ureaplasma carriers,* however, contain few or no PMN leukocytes and the distribution of generally low numbers of *Ureaplasma* colonies in such controls, is random. Thus, the frequent, close association of ureaplasmas with urinary mucous threads from men with NGU further supports an etiological role in this disease.

Quantitative studies

If ureaplasmas are one of the etiologic agents of NGU, it should be possible to demonstrate culturally a close, *quantitative* relationship between the organism and the clinical events of the disease. This was first accomplished in 1974 by SHEPARD (17) who performed quantitative cultures of urine specimens collected *daily,* before, during and following treatment of *Ureaplasma*-positive NGU patients with deliberately low regimens of tetracyclines. Thirty-two NGU patients were treated with only 2 to 4 g of tetracyclines over three to four days time. Of the 23 treated patients who were successfully followed, 12 were cured, and 2 failed treatment. However, *9 patients* experienced both clinical and ureaplasmal relapse following an eclipse period without symptoms of 8 to 45 days (mean = 22 ± 11 days).

Quantitative studies were also reported by BOWIE et al. (5) who found a strong association between chlamydia-negative NGU and ureaplasmas. *U. urealyticum* was the only agent found to be significantly associated with chlamydia-negative NGU, and first voided urine titers of 10^3, 10^4, and 10^5 organisms were considered to be etiologically important. WEIDNER et al. (28), in a quantitative study of 312 men with prostato-urethritis, and WEIDNER et al. (27), in a quantitative study of 187 men with chronic prostatitis and 108 healthy controls, found ureaplasma titers from 10^3 to 10^5 CFU/ml in prostatic fluid and urine specimens to be etiologically significant.

Human inoculation studies

A pathogenic role for ureaplasmas in NGU is more firmly established by the carefully controlled, experimental inoculation study of human volunteers conducted by TAYLOR-ROBINSON et al. (25). These authors reported the production of *clinical urethritis* in two human volunteers who were inoculated intraurethrally with purified, serotype 5 ureaplasmas recently isolated from men with chlamydia-negative NGU. Both subjects developed urethritis characterized by dysuria, frequency, urethral discharge, discomfort and pyuria. Both subjects developed a rise in serum antibody titer of 1:16; in one subject the titer persisted at 1:8,3 months after inoculation. Following treatment with tetracycline, signs and symptoms disappeared and ureaplasmas were eliminated. JÄNSCH (11) was the first to inoculate a human volunteer with a pure culture of ureaplasmas, but details of source, age, purification, numbers of organisms inoculated, and freedom from chlamydia, were not reported. Three days after inoculation, the subject developed urethritis with dysuria and urethral discharge. Large numbers of ureaplasmas were isolated from the urethral exudate. Following doxycycline therapy, the urethritis subsided and the ureaplasmas were eliminated. These human inoculation studies clearly establish that ureaplasmas are pathogenic for the male genital tract, and there is no reason to doubt that certain ureaplasma strains are capable of causing urethritis in man.

Response to certain selective antibiotics

The use of selective or differential antibiotics has also proved useful in resolving the role of ureaplasmas in genital tract infections. BOWIE et al. (1, 3) reported that NGU persisted in men not only after treatment with sulfafurazole — which eliminated chlamydia but not ureaplasmas — but also after treatment with aminocyclitols (spectinomycin & streptomycin), which eradicated ureaplasmas but not chlamydia. These findings suggested that *both* organisms were important as a cause of NGU. COUFALIK et al. (6) reached similar conclusions in a double-blind therapeutic trial of minocycline and rifampicin on men with NGU. Minocycline is effective against both chlamydia and ureaplasmas, whereas ureaplasmas are unaffected by rifampicin and fail to be eradicated by the drug. It was also observed that Reiter's syndrome developed in two men treated with rifampicin from whom only ureaplasmas were isolated initially.

Tetracycline resistance

Ford and Smith (9) first reported the isolation of a tetracycline-resistant strain of *U. urealyticum* from an NGU patient whose urethritis was unaffected by treatment with tetracycline, 500 mg 3 times daily for 5 days. The patient subsequently responded to retreatment with a different drug, erythromycin, to which the organism was *sensitive.* Cultures for chlamydia regrettably were not performed. The ureaplasma strain was resistant to about 20 times the concentration of tetracycline that inhibited stock ureaplasma strains. Other authors have since reported the isolation of tetracycline-resistant ureaplasmas from individuals with genital tract infection. Spaepen et al. (21) isolated tetracycline-resistant ureaplasmas from women with a history of reproductive failure, and estimated that from 6 to 10% or more of ureaplasma strains are now tetracycline-resistant. Evans et al. (7) reported that 10% of ureaplasma isolates were resistant to tetracycline, and that all of them were sensitive to erythromycin. Repeated passages increased the resistance to minocycline of three out of four strains.

Persistent NGU due to tetracycline-resistant ureaplasmas

The recent emergence of tetracycline-resistant strains of *U. urealyticum* provides an excellent opportunity to further examine the etiologic role of this organism in genital tract disease. Two separate studies [Bowie et al. (2); Stimson et al. (22)] report the isolation of tetracycline-resistant ureaplasmas from chlamydia-negative men with NGU who were unresponsive to treatment with tetracycline. These NGU patients were successfully treated and cured *only* when they were retreated with a different drug to which the ureaplasmas were sensitive (erythromycin). Tetracycline resistance was significantly correlated with the persistence of ureaplasmas, and persistence of NGU during treatment. Similar observations have been made in 14 chlamydia-negative NGU patients from whom tetracycline-resistant ureaplasmas were isolated by Brown (unpublished observation).

Conclusion

There is now mounting, convincing evidence that *Ureaplasma urealyticum* is a human pathogen. Additional evidence is provided by more recent controlled isolation studies, including studies of chlamydia-negative men with NGU, the association of ureaplasmas with urinary mucous threads in men with NGU, quantitative studies, the differential response of chlamydia and ureaplasmas to certain antibiotics, human inoculation studies, and the emergence of tetracy-cline-resistant ureaplasmas associated with persistent NGU in chlamydia-negative men. All this suggests that *Ureaplasma urealyticum* is an important cause of genital tract disease in man.

References

(1) Bowie, W. R., S.-P. Wang, E. R. Alexander, K. K. Holmes: Etiology of nongonococcal urethritis. In: Hobson, D., K. K. Holmes (eds.): Nongonococcal urethritis and related infections; pp. 19–29. American Society for Microbiology, Washington, D. C. 1977.

(2) Bowie, W. R., J. S. Yu, A. Fawcett, H. D. Jones: Tetracycline in nongonococcal urethritis: comparison of 2 g and 1 g daily for seven days. Brit. J. Vener. Dis. *56*: 332–336 (1980).

(3) Bowie, W. R., E. R. Alexander, J. F. Floyd, J. Holmes, Y. Miller, K. K. Holmes: Differential response of chlamydial and ureaplasma-associated urethritis to sulfafurazole (sulfisoxazole) and aminocyclitols. Lancet *II*: 1276–1278 (1976).

(4) Bowie, W. R., H. M. Pollock, P. S. Forsyth, J. F. Floyd, E. R. Alexander, S.-P. Wang, K. K. Holmes: Bacteriology of the urethra in normal men and men with nongonococcal urethritis. J. Clin. Microbiol. *6*: 482–488 (1977).

(5) Bowie, W. R., S.-P. Wang, E. R. Alexander, J. Floyd, P. S. Forsyth, H. M. Pollock, J.-S. L. Lin, T. M. Buchanan, K. K. Holmes: Etiology of nongonococcal urethritis: evidence for Chlamydia trachomatis and Ureaplasma urealyticum. J. Clin. Invest. *59*: 735–742 (1977).

(6) Coufalik, E. D., D. Taylor-Robinson, G. W. Csonka: Treatment of nongonococcal urethritis with rifampicin as a means of defining the role of Ureaplasma urealyticum. Brit. J. Vener. Dis. *55*: 36–43 (1979).

(7) Evans, R. T., D. Taylor-Robinson: Incidence of tetracycline-resistant strains of Ureaplasma urealyticum. J. Antimicrob. Chemother. *4*: 57–64 (1978).

(8) Fodor, M.: Difference in the virulence of Ureaplasma urealyticum isolates. Acta microbiologica Acad. Sci. hung. *27*: 161–169 (1980).

(9) Ford, D. K., J. R. Smith: Non-specific urethritis associated with a tetracycline-resistant T-mycoplasma. Brit. J. Vener. Dis. *50*: 373–374 (1974).

(10) Howard, C. J., R. N. Gourlay, J. Brownlie: The virulence of T-mycoplasma, isolated from various animal species, assayed by intramammary inoculation in cattle. J. Hyg. (Camb.) *71*: 163–170 (1973).

(11) Jänsch, H. H.: Pathogenitätsnachweis für harnstoffspaltende Mycoplasmen im menschlichen Urogenitaltrakt im Selbstversuch. Hautarzt *23*: 558 (1972).

(12) McCormack, W. M., Y.-H. Lee, S. H. Zinner: Sexual experience and urethral colonization with genital mycoplasmas: a study in normal men. Ann. Int. Med. *78*: 696–698 (1973).

(13) Millar, J. W., E. E. Siess, H. A. Feldman, C. Silverman, P. Frank: In vivo and in vitro resistance to sulfadiazine in strains of Neisseria meningitidis. J. Am. Med. Assn. *186*: 139–141 (1963).

(14) Shepard, M. C.: The recovery of pleuropneumonia-like organisms from Negro men with and without nongonococcal urethritis. Am. J. Syph. Gonorrhea Vener. Dis. *38*: 113–124 (1954).

(15) Shepard, M. C.: Non-gonococcal urethritis in the Camp Lejeune area. Urol. Intern. *9*: 252–257 (1959).

(16) Shepard, M. C.: Nongonococcal urethritis associated with human strains of „T" mycoplasmas. J. Am. Med. Assn. *211*: 1335–1340 (1970).

(17) SHEPARD, M. C.: Quantitative relationship of Ureaplasma urealyticum to the clinical course of nongonococcal urethritis in the human male. Colloque de L'Institut National de la Santé et de la Recherche Médicale, Bordeaux, France, Les mycoplasmes. INSERM *33*: 375−380 (1974).

(18) SHEPARD, M. C.: Ureaplasma urealyticum in urinary mucous threads from male nongonococcal urethritis patients. Zbl. Bakt. Hyg., I. Abt. Orig. A *241*: 271 (1978).

(19) SHEPARD, M. C., R. S. COMBS: Enhancement of Ureaplasma urealyticum growth on a differential agar medium (A7B) by a polyamine, putrescine. J. Clin. Microbiol. *10*: 931−933 (1979).

(20) SHEPARD, M. C., C. D. LUNCEFORD: Differential agar medium (A7) for identification of Ureaplasma urealyticum (human T mycoplasmas) in primary cultures of clinical material. J. Clin. Microbiol. *3*: 613−625 (1976).

(21) SPAEPEN, M. S., R. B. KUNDSIN, H. W. HORNE: Tetracycline-resistant T-mycoplasmas (Ureaplasma urealyticum) from patients with a history of reproductive failure. Antimicrob. Agents Chemother. *9*: 1012−1013 (1976).

(22) STIMSON, J. B., J. HALE, W. R. BOWIE, K. K. HOLMES: Tetracycline-resistant Ureaplasma urealyticum: a cause of persistent nongonococcal urethritis. Ann. Int. Med. *94*: 192−194 (1981).

(23) TAYLOR-ROBINSON, D., W. M. MCCORMACK: Mycoplasmas in human genitourinary infections. In: TULLY, J. G., R. F. WHITCOMB (eds.): The mycoplasmas. Vol. II: Human and animal mycoplasmas; pp. 307−366. Academic Press, New York 1979.

(24) TAYLOR-ROBINSON, D., W. M. MCCORMACK: The genital mycoplasmas. New Engl. J. Med. *302*: 1003−1010; 1063−1067 (1980).

(25) TAYLOR-ROBINSON, D., G. W. CSONKA, M. J. PRENTICE: Human intra-urethral inoculation of ureaplasmas. Quart. J. Med. (New Series) *46*: 309−326 (1977).

(26) TAYLOR-ROBINSON, D., R. T. EVANS, E. D. COUFALIK, M. J. PRENTICE, P. E. MUNDAY, G. W. CSONKA, J. K. OATES: Ureaplasma urealyticum and Mycoplasma hominis in chlamydial and non-chlamydial nongonococcal urethritis. Brit. J. Vener. Dis. *55*: 30−35 (1979).

(27) WEIDNER, W., H. BRUNNER, W. KRAUSE: Quantitative culture of Ureaplasma urealyticum in patients with chronic prostatitis or prostatosis. J. Urol. *124*: 622−625 (1980).

(28) WEIDNER, W., H. BRUNNER, W. KRAUSE, C. F. ROTHAUGE: Zur Bedeutung von Ureaplasma urealyticum bei unspezifischer Prostato-Urethritis. Quantitative Untersuchungen an 312 Patienten. Dtsch. med. Wschr. *103*: 465−470 (1978).

(29) WONG, J. L., P. A. HINES, M. D. BRASHER, G. T. ROGERS, R. F. SMITH, J. SCHACHTER: The etiology of nongonococcal urethritis in men attending a venereal disease clinic. Sex. Trans. Dis. *5*: 4−8 (1977).

Division of Communicable Diseases, MRC Clinical Research Centre, Harrow, Middlesex

Microbiological Aspects of Non-Gonococcal Urethro-Prostatitis and its Probable Consequences

D. TAYLOR-ROBINSON, P. E. MUNDAY, N. F. HANNA, B. J. THOMAS, P. M. FURR

Non-gonococcal urethritis and infection of the prostate

There is considerable evidence that *Chlamydia trachomatis* organisms (chlamydiae) are a cause of acute non-gonococcal urethritis (NGU) (TAYLOR-ROBINSON and THOMAS, 1980) and evidence also that *Ureaplasma urealyticum* organisms (ureaplasmas) are responsible for some cases of this disease (TAYLOR-ROBINSON and CSONKA, 1981). Examination of expressed prostatic secretion in a patient who has NGU is, of course, insufficient to determine whether the prostate is infected because inevitably the secretion will be "contaminated" by organisms in the urethra. More sophisticated procedures are required which are often beyond the scope of the routine procedures of venereology departments and the problem comes within the realm of a research investigation. Our studies have not been designed to determine the proportion of patients suffering from NGU who also have involvement of the prostate, although we surmise that many of them have a prostatic infection, if not prostatic disease. This supposition is fortified by the results of detailed observations made on one of two volunteers who were inoculated intraurethrally with ureaplasmas (TAYLOR-ROBINSON et al., 1977). In addition to urethritis, there was evidence of urea-plasmal infection of the prostate. This conclusion was based on the finding that the largest number of organisms occurred in the prostatic portion of fraction-ated semen samples. Determining whether there is chlamydial infection of the prostate by this or other quantitative procedures would be more difficult; urine and secretions are often toxic for cell monolayers used in the isolation proce-dure and, furthermore, there is some evidence that prostatic and seminal fluids may adversely affect the isolation of chlamydiae (MÅRDH, personal communi-cation).

Complications of NGU

The possible complications of acute NGU or urethro-prostatitis are persistent or recurrent urethritis, acute epididymitis, chronic urethro-prostatitis, and sexually acquired reactive arthritis (SARA), including Reiter's disease. These complications and the problem of infertility are discussed.

Persistent and recurrent urethritis

There is no doubt that acute NGU is not always an easily curable disease and persistence and recurrence may be regarded, perhaps, as part of the natural history of the disease rather than complications. In a clinical and microbiological study of 221 male patients with NGU (MUNDAY et al., 1981; MUNDAY et al., 1982) follow-up examinations were continued until patients were cured or until they defaulted. Many patients had symptoms and signs of persistent or recurrent disease after treatment with minocycline. Thus, only 79 patients (36%) responded as expected and were discharged cured early in the study. At the end of the study, 98 patients (44%) had been discharged cured, 50 (23%) had defaulted when cured and 72 (33%) were not cured when last seen. The clinical outcome in relation to the initial microbiological findings is shown in Table 1. The cure rates at one week, one month and at the end of the study were broadly similar, taking into account the increasing proportion of defaulting patients as the study progressed. Furthermore, the clinical outcome of patients in most microbiological groups was similar, although the lowest cure rate throughout the study was seen in those who were infected with chlamydiae and mycoplasmas (C+M+). A large proportion of patients defaulted in this group but 26% were still attending at one month which suggests that their disease was persistent. Although this may be due occasionally to the persistence of tetracycline-resistant ureaplasmas (STIMSON et al., 1981), we found such organ-

Table 1. NGU cure rates in relation to the initial microbiological diagnosis.
(Data from MUNDAY et al., 1981 and 1982.)

| Microbiological | Cure rate (%) at | | |
diagnosis	1 week	1 month	end of study
C+ M−	53	60	61
C+ M+	44	23	26
C− M+	55	39	42
C− M−	45	36	42

isms in patients without disease as frequently as in those with disease. However, re-infection by recognised pathogens occurred rarely and the possibility that aberrant immunological mechanisms are responsible for persistent disease needs investigation. WESTON (1965) suggested an allergic basis for NGU, and the possibility that atopic patients are more likely to develop persistent disease needs careful study.

The severe response to a primary chlamydial infection of the urethra was observed following intra-urethral inoculation of chimpanzees (TAYLOR-ROBINSON et al., 1981). We were fortunate to be able to examine histological sections of the urethra of one of these animals three months after inoculation. At this time, that is two months after the animal had been treated with a tetracycline and chlamydiae were not recoverable, the submucosal region was densely infiltrated with small round cells, presumably lymphocytes. One may surmise that the same phenomenon occurs in man.

Chronic urethro-prostatitis

The prostate may harbour micro-organisms in patients who have persistent symptoms and signs following an acute attack of NGU. Of 217 patients with NGU who were studied (COUFALIK et al., 1979), 28 developed persistent symptoms and signs of urethritis and prostatitis in spite of multiple courses of various antibiotics over a two-year period. During this time up to 15 isolation attempts were made, but chlamydiae were not isolated and ureaplasmas were isolated only rarely from the anterior urethra, sometimes after prostatic massage. Because of their problems, eleven of the patients volunteered to have a detailed examination in hospital. It is interesting that on admission, ureaplasmas were isolated from the anterior urethra of five of them, three of whom harboured also *Mycoplasma hominis*. Six patients were apparently free of all these micro-organisms, but ureaplasmas were isolated from four of them, one of whom also had *M. hominis,* when secretions were obtained by introducing a catheter into the prostatic urethra followed by prostatic massage (COULFALIK, TAYLOR-ROBINSON and FURR, unpublished observations). In all chronic disease conditions, however, the isolation of a micro-organism long after the disease began may not mean that it was responsible for initiating the disease and it is mere speculation that the ureaplasmas and/or *M. hominis* were responsible for perpetuating the condition. Whether antibody studies, particularly on prostatic secretions, would be of help in establishing a relationship between genital micro-organisms and this chronic disease is debatable. However, such studies would seem worthwhile in view of the success of the serological approach in the case of Reiter's disease.

Acute epididymitis

One group of investigators (HARNISCH et al., 1977) suggested that ureaplasmas might cause epididymitis. However, the results of subsequent studies by the same workers (BERGER et al., 1978) failed to support their hypothesis. Although many of the men with unexplained epididymitis had ureaplasmal organisms in the urethra, only one man had more than 10^3 organisms and no ureaplasmas were recovered from percutaneous aspirates of the inflamed epididymis. These investigators concluded that in men under 35 years of age most cases of epididymitis are due to *N. gonorrhoeae* or chlamydiae, whereas in older men gram-negative bacilli are usually responsible. Further studies of this kind are desirable although many workers may not deem it appropriate to take epididymal aspirates.

Sexually acquired reactive arthritis (SARA) and Reiter's disease

The problems encountered in determining the cause of chronic disease in the male genital tract are not dissimilar from those seen in establishing the cause of arthritis which develops in about 1% of men with acute NGU or urethro-prostatitis.

To attempt to associate arthritis with infection in the genital tract months after the arthritis has developed is a hopeless task. Furthermore, since arthritis occurs often after patients have been treated for NGU with tetracyclines, microbiological investigation is likely to be unrewarding. However, KEAT et al. (1980) examined untreated patients with arthritis soon after the development of urethritis and found that 43% of them had evidence of a chlamydial genital infection; this was based on the isolation of chlamydiae from the urethra and/or the presence of chlamydial IgM antibody measured by micro-immunofluorescence (IMF).

This chlamydial infection rate was little different from that found in patients with uncomplicated NGU and was an insufficient reason to incriminate the organisms as a cause of the arthritis, particularly since viable chlamydiae have not been found in the joints (THOMAS, unpublished data). However, the chlamydial IgG IMF antibody responses in the patients with arthritis were much greater (mean titre: 1 in 47.5) than in those with uncomplicated NGU (mean titre: 1 in 8.6) and, indeed, antibody titres were greater in the sera of the SARA patients than in those of patients with a variety of other arthritides. It would seem reasonable to propose that genital chlamydial infection is a triggering factor in the development of arthritis in about half the patients but the exact mechanism whereby it develops is unknown: it would seem to be a truly reactive arthritis because there is, as yet, no evidence of joint infection.

The results of further studies on patients presenting to a venereology clinic with urethritis and arthritis (HANNA, THOMAS and TAYLOR-ROBINSON, unpublished observations) have underlined, first, the impossibility of isolating chlamydiae once a patient has been treated with a tetracycline or erythromycin, and second, the occurrence of high titres of chlamydial IMF antibody most often in patients with clear-cut evidence of Reiter's disease. Further, ureaplasmas were found frequently in the absence of chlamydiae, but no more often in patients with Reiter's disease than in those with arthralgia, other arthritides or in those without evidence of joint disease. However, to determine whether ureaplasmas have any role in Reiter's disease and whether they might, in particular, have any involvement in non-chlamydial disease, it will be necessary to undertake serological tests to determine whether antibody responses to these organisms are exaggerated in a way similar to that seen for chlamydiae. It would be unwise at this stage to discount ureaplasmas completely for we know that they have arthritogenic potential; in patients with hypogammaglobulinaemia they have been found to cause septic arthritis (TAYLOR-ROBINSON, 1981).

Infertility

Spermatozoa adsorb to colonies and suspensions of certain mycoplasmas, including some strains of ureaplasmas. This adsorption has raised the question of whether mycoplasmas, particularly ureaplasmas, might cause infertility in men. O'Leary and his colleagues have conducted several studies concerned with the association of ureaplasmas with male infertility (O'LEARY and FRICK, 1975; FOWLKES et al., 1975; TOTH et al., 1978; SWENSON et al., 1979) and have reported that semen samples containing ureaplasmas had poorer motility, fewer spermatozoa and more aberrant forms than did samples without ureaplasmas. Successful treatment of ureaplasmal infection was associated with improvement in spermatozoal motility and a decrease in certain abnormal features of seminal cytology. Other workers (HOFSTETTER et al., 1978) have also linked ureaplasmas to abnormalities of spermatozoa, but DESAI et al. (1980) and ourselves (TAYLOR-ROBINSON and FURR, 1973; TAYLOR-ROBINSON and FURR, unpublished data: see Table 2) have not been able to do so.

TRAUB et al. (1973) attempted to isolate mycoplasmas from the vas deferens taken at vasectomy but were unsuccessful. Likewise, we (TAYLOR-ROBINSON and FURR, unpublished data) examined vas deferens specimens taken at vasectomy from men attending a family planning clinic. Semen samples from 33 of

Table 2. Isolation of ureaplasmas from human seminal fluids. (Data of TAYLOR-ROBINSON and FURR, unpublished.)

Fertility	No. of persons	No. of fluids with indicated no. of CCU[a]/ml							% isolation
		Nil	10^1	10^2	10^3	10^4	10^5	10^6	
Normal	14	6			4 (3)[b]	2	1	1 (1)	57
Borderline	9	4			4 (3)	1 (1)			55
Low	28	9	1	1	8 (6)	6 (3)	2 (1)	1	68
Known fertile	3		1	1	1 (1)				67

[a]   CCU = colour-changing units.
[b]   ( )   = those specimens in which 10% or more of the ureaplasmas were adherent.

the men before vasectomy contained ureaplasmas and six of these also contained *M. hominis,* but none of the vas deferens specimens contained these organisms. There is no information of the same kind about infertile men, or men with overt genital-tract disease, although it is interesting to note that BERGER et al. (1978) did not isolate ureaplasmas from percutaneous aspirates of the epididymis taken from 16 patients with acute epididymitis. It seems unlikely, therefore, that many infertile men have ureaplasmas in the vas deferens and it is likely that ureaplasmas in their semen gain entrance from the urethra or prostate at the time of ejaculation. It would be surprising, therefore, if these organisms could affect spermatogenesis. Furthermore, because of the probable time of ureaplasmal access to semen, and in view of the small number of organisms relative to the number of spermatozoa (usually no more than 1 organism: 10 spermatozoa) even in a sample of "infertile" semen, it would be remarkable if these organisms could appreciably affect motility in a freshly collected specimen. There are no data relevant to chlamydial infection and male infertility probably because the designing of such a study poses even greater problems than those concerned with ureaplasmas. Although singling out specific micro-organisms and attempting to examine their role in male infertility is perhaps a valid approach, the extent to which attacks of NGU and its subsequent complications may affect male fertility seems to be unknown. Studies designed to answer this question would appear to be relatively straightforward and worthwhile.

A newly discovered mycoplasma

The isolation of a mycoplasma, distinct from all others, from the urethra of men with NGU has been recorded recently (TULLY et al., 1981; TAYLOR-ROBINSON et al., 1981). This organism has the appearance and adsorptive capacity usually associated with pathogenic mycoplasmas. Whether it could cause any of the non-chlamydial, non-ureaplasmal cases of NGU or, indeed, be implicated in any of the complications mentioned above deserves attention.

References

(1) BERGER, R. E., E. R. ALEXANDER, G. D. MONDA, J. ANSELL, G. McCORMICK, K. K. HOLMES: Chlamydia trachomatis as a cause of acute „idiopathic" epididymitis. New Engl. J. Med. *298*: 301–304 (1978).

(2) COUFALIK, E. D., D. TAYLOR-ROBINSON, G. W. CSONKA: Treatment of nongonococcal urethritis with rifampicin as a means of defining the role of Ureaplasma urealyticum. Brit. J. Ven. Dis. *55*: 36–43 (1979).

(3) DESAI, S., M. S. COHEN, M. KHATAMEE, E. LEITER: Ureaplasma urealyticum (T-mycoplasma) infection: does it have a role in male infertility? J. Urol. *124*: 469–471 (1980).

(4) FOWLKES, D. M., J. MACLEOD, W. M. O'LEARY: T-mycoplasmas and human infertility: correlation of infection with alterations in seminal parameters. Fertil. Steril. *26*: 1212–1218 (1975).

(5) HARNISCH, J. P., R. E. BERGER, E. R. ALEXANDER, G. MONDA, K. K. HOLMES: Aetiology of acute epididymitis. Lancet *1*: 819–821 (1977).

(6) HOFSTETTER, A., E. SCHMIEDT, W.-B. SCHILL, H. H. WOLFF: Genitale Mykoplasmenstämme als Ursache der männlichen Infertilität. Helv. Chir. Acta. *45*: 329–333 (1978).

(7) KEAT, A. C., B. J. THOMAS, D. TAYLOR-ROBINSON, G. D. PEGRUM, R. N. MAINI, J. T. SCOTT: Evidence of Chlamydia trachomatis infection in sexually acquired reactive arthritis. Ann. Rheum. Dis. *39*: 431–437 (1980).

(8) MUNDAY, P. E., B. J. THOMAS, A. P. JOHNSON, D. G. ALTMAN, D. TAYLOR-ROBINSON: Clinical and microbiological study of non-gonococcal urethritis with particular reference to non-chlamydial disease. Brit. J. Ven. Dis. *57*: 327–333 (1981).

(9) MUNDAY, P. E., D. G. ALTMAN, A. P. JOHNSON, B. J. THOMAS, D. TAYLOR-ROBINSON: Persistent and recurrent non-gonococcal urethritis without evidence of current infection. Europ. J. Sex. Trans. Dis. *1*: 15–20 (1982).

(10) O'LEARY, W. M., J. FRICK: The correlation of human male infertility with the presence of mycoplasma T-strains. Andrologia *7*: 309–316 (1975).

(11) STIMSON, J. B., J. HALE, W. R. BOWIE, K. K. HOLMES: Tetracycline-resistant Ureaplasma urealyticum: a cause of persistent nongonococcal urethritis. Ann. Intern. Med. *94*: 192–194 (1981).

(12) SWENSON, C. E., A. TOTH, W. M. O'LEARY: Ureaplasma urealyticum and human infertility: the effect of antibiotic therapy on semen quality. Fertil. Steril. *31*: 660–665 (1979).

(13) TAYLOR-ROBINSON, D.: Mycoplasmal arthritis in man. Israel J. Med. Sci. *17*: 616–621 (1981).

(14) TAYLOR-ROBINSON, D., G. W. CSONKA: Laboratory and clinical aspects of mycoplasmal infections of the human genitourinary tract. In: HARRIS, J. R. W. (ed.): Recent Advances in Sexually Transmitted Diseases; pp. 151–186. Churchill Livingstone, London 1981.

(15) TAYLOR-ROBINSON, D., G. W. CSONKA, M. J. PRENTICE: Human intra-urethral inoculation of ureaplasmas. Quart. J. Med. *46*: 309–326 (1977).

(16) Taylor-Robinson, D., R. H. Purcell, W. T. London, D. L. Sly, B. J. Thomas, R. T. Evans: Microbiological, serological and histopathological features of experimental Chlamydia trachomatis urethritis in chimpanzees. Brit. J. Ven. Dis. *57*: 36—40 (1981).

(17) Taylor-Robinson, D., B. J. Thomas: The role of Chlamydia trachomatis in genital-tract and associated diseases. J. Clin. Path. *33*: 205—233 (1980).

(18) Taylor-Robinson, D., J. G. Tully, P. M. Furr, R. M. Cole, D. L. Rose, N. F. Hanna: Urogenital mycoplasma infections of man: a review with observations on a recently discovered mycoplasma. Israel J. Med. Sci. *17*: 524—530 (1981).

(19) Toth, A., C. E. Swenson, W. M. O'Leary: Light microscopy as an aid in predicting ureaplasma infection in human semen. Fertil. Steril. *30*: 586—591 (1978).

(20) Traub, R. G., D. L. Madden, D. A. Fuccillo, T. W. McLean: The male as a reservoir of infection with cytomegalovirus, herpes and mycoplasma. New Engl. J. Med. *289*: 697—698 (1973).

(21) Tully, J. G., D. Taylor-Robinson, R. M. Cole, D. L. Rose: A newly discovered mycoplasma in the human urogenital tract. Lancet *1*: 1288—1291 (1981).

(22) Weston, T. E. T.: An allergic basis for non-specific urethritis. Brit. J. Ven. Dis. *41*: 107—116 (1965).

Department of Medical Microbiology and Regional Public Health Laboratory,
St. Elisabeth Ziekenhuis, Tilburg
National Institute of Public Health, Bilthoven
Department of Urology, St. Radboud Ziekenhuis, University of Nijmegen
Department of Medical Microbiology, St. Radboud Ziekenhuis, University of Nijmegen

Abacterial Prostatitis: Microbiological Data

M. Peeters, A. Polak-Vogelzang, F. Debruyne, J. van der Veen

Introduction

In only a minority of cases of clinically diagnosed chronic prostatitis can pathogenic bacteria be found in the prostatic secretion. In most instances, normal bacteriological cultures of prostatic fluid remain sterile even in the presence of a nearly purulent prostatic secretion. The majority of cases are therefore considered to be due to non-bacterial causes.

Since in many patients with symptoms of chronic prostatitis no known uro-genital tract pathogens can be isolated (and in addition no increase of leuco-cytes in the prostatic fluid is found) it is questionable whether an infection is always the cause of this condition. Many clinicians consider the symptoms of a substantial number of these patients to be psychological rather than somatic in origin.

In our study the role of various micro-organisms in the pathogenesis of chronic prostatitis was investigated.

Materials and Methods

Specimens were examined from 102 patients with symptoms and signs of chronic prostatitis, which had been present for at least 3 months. The patients varied in age from 18 to 69 years, and the mean age was 40.

Urethral samples (taken with a sterile loop), the first 10 ml of voided urine, the midstream-portion of urine, prostatic fluid (expressed by massage) and the first 10 ml of urine after prostatic massage were collected from each patient. One week later seminal fluid obtained by masturbation was received. All speci-mens were incubated on blood agar plates under aerobic and anaerobic condi-tions and further tested for *Neisseria gonorrhoeae, yeasts, Trichomonas vagi-*

nalis, Mycoplasma hominis, Ureaplasma urealyticum, Chlamydia trachomatis, herpes simplex-virus, and cytomegalovirus.

For cultivating *N. gonorrhoeae* TM-medium was used (THAYER and MARTIN, 1966), for yeasts Sabouraud dextrose agar and for *T. vaginalis* a casein hydrolysate-serum medium (LASH, 1950). For cultivating and identifying *M. hominis* and *U. urealyticum* we used trypticase soy broth-urea U9 medium (SHEPARD and LUNCEFORD, 1970), Differential agar medium A7 (SHEPARD and LUNCEFORD, 1976), and Herderscheê-medium (HERDERSCHEÊ, 1963). Because serotypes of Ureaplasma may differ in pathogenicity (SHEPARD and LUNCEFORD, 1978), all isolated strains were serotyped by means of indirect immunofluorescence (BLACK and KROGSGAARD-JENSEN, 1974; PANANGALA and LEIN, 1978). For isolation of *C. trachomatis* diethylaminoethyl-dextran and cycloheximide-treated HeLa-229 cells were used (CROY et al., 1975; KUO et al., 1977).

To point out the presence of virus the specimens were inoculated into human embryonic lung fibroblast tissue cultures and the cultures were observed for 6 weeks for any cytopathogenic effect before being discarded (LENNETTE and SMIDT, 1969). Serum specimens from the patients were tested for antibodies to Chlamydia by means of a micro-immunofluorescence test (WANG and GRAYSTON, 1974) and for antibodies against herpes simplex-virus and cytomegalovirus by means of the complement-fixation test.

The results were compared with those obtained from a group of 51 healthy men, varying in age from 27 to 52 years, whose mean age was 38 years. These 51 men were subjected to the same procedures, except for prostatic massage. There were two reasons for omitting the massage:
1. It is very difficult to find a volunteer for such a procedure which is painful.
2. It is seldom possible to obtain prostatic fluid from a healthy person.

The prostates of the patients are mostly congested and this makes it possible to press out fluid in most cases. The omittence of tests of prostatic fluid in control persons was probably not a serious shortcoming, because one of the results of the study of the patients was that seminal fluid is a good alternative for prostatic fluid in microbiological study.

Results

In 15 of the 102 patients aerobic bacteria were found to be the cause of the illness (11 *E. coli*, 2 *Staphylococcus aureus*, 1 *Klebsiella pneumoniae*, 1 *Neisseria gonorrhoeae*). The bacteria were present in prostatic fluid as well as in seminal fluid in counts of approximately 100,000 per ml. In most cases there was a positive antibody-coating. Thus, approximately 15% of the patients had chronic prostatitis due to bacteria.

In one of our patients *Trichomonas vaginalis* and in another a yeast *(Torulopsis glabrata)* was found to be the cause of the illness.

In one patient with bacterial prostatitis herpes simplex-virus was isolated, in two patients cytomegalovirus (in these two cases the viruses disappeared spontaneously without any change in the patients condition). There were no significant differences in the antibody titers against herpes simplex-virus and cytomegalovirus between patients and healthy men.

Anaerobic bacteria were isolated from the urethral samples and the seminal fluid from more then half of the patients and healthy controls (mostly peptococci, peptostreptococci, Veillonella and Bacteroides) but always in very low counts. A pure culture of anaerobes in prostatic or seminal fluid was never found in counts exceeding 10,000 per ml.

The overall results shown in Table 1 indicate that only 17 of the 102 patients had prostatitis due to known urogenital tract pathogens and that 85 had "non-specific"[1] prostatitis.

Mycoplasma hominis was found in 2 healthy controls and 11 patients. When only "non-specific" cases were considered, it appeared that 10 of the 85 cases were positive for mycoplasmas.

Table 1. Number of patients with prostatitis due to known urogenital tract pathogens (n = 102).

Bacteria	15 (11 E. coli, 2 Staphylococcus aureus, 1 Klebsiella pneumoniae, 1 Neisseria gonorrhoeae)
Trichomonas	1
Yeasts	1 (Torulopsis glabrata)
Total	17 (16.6%)

Table 2. Frequency of isolations of Mycoplasma and Ureaplasma from healthy controls and patients.

Mycoplasma hominis:	
2/ 51 healthy controls	(3.9%)
11/102 patients	(10.8%) (p = 0.26)
10/ 85 patients with "non-specific" prostatitis	(11.8%) (p = 0.21)
Ureaplasma urealyticum:	
13/ 51 healthy controls	(25.5%)
42/102 patients	(41.2%) (p = 0.08)
40/ 85 patients with "non-specific" prostatitis	(47.1%) (p = 0.02)

---

[1] The term "non-specific" is used here in the sense of "not caused by known pathogens".

Table 3. Frequency of isolations of Mycoplasma, Ureaplasma or Chlamydia, alone and of combinations of these agents from patients with "non-specific" prostatitis and from healthy controls.

Organisms isolated	Patients (n = 85)	Healthy controls (n = 51)
Mycoplasma hominis	2	1
Ureaplasma urealyticum	30	12
M. hominis + U. urealyticum	8	1
Chlamydia trachomatis	5	0
C. trachomatis + U. urealyticum	2	0
Only "commensal" flora*	38	37

* i.c. diphtheroids, *Staph. epidermidis*, micrococci, α-streptococci, peptococci, peptostreptococci.

Table 4. Antibodies against *C. trachomatis* in the microimmunofluorence test in patients with chronic prostatitis and healthy controls.

Titer	No. of patients (n = 102)		No. of healthy controls (n = 51)	
<1:8	52	(51%)	42	(82.4%)
1:8	9		1	
1:16	16		3	
1:32	10	(49%)	3	(17.6%)
1:64	7		1	
1:128	6		1	
>1:128	2		0	

Ureaplasma urealyticum was isolated from 13 (25.5%) of the 51 healthy controls and from 42 (41.2%) of the 102 patients. When we considered only the 85 cases of "non-specific" prostatitis, it appeared that 40 (47%) of the 85 were positive for Ureaplasma. This difference in isolation rates between patients with "non-specific" prostatitis and healthy controls was significant (Table 2).

Table 3 shows the frequency of isolations of Mycoplasma, Ureaplasma or Chlamydia alone and of combinations of these agents from patients with "non-specific" prostatitis and for healthy controls. From 38 patients only commensal flora could be isolated.

The serological study showed that 50 (49%) of the patients had antibodies to Chlamydia (titer ≥ 1:8), in contrast to 9 (18%) of the 51 controls. This difference was highly significant (p = 0.0003) (Table 4).

All patients with "non-specific" prostatitis associated with *M. hominis* (2), *U. urealyticum* (30), *M. hominis* + *U. urealyticum* (8), *C. trachomatis* (5) and *C. trachomatis* + *U. urealyticum* (2) were treated with tetracycline (1,000 mg per day) or doxycycline (100 mg per day) for 25 days. The sexual partners were also treated during the same time. The organisms disappeared from all (2 patients needed 2 cures) and 12 patients with *U. urealyticum* (2 + *M. hominis*) became free of symptoms (Table 5). These 12 patients had high leucocyte counts in their prostatic fluid or urine after prostatic massage, and these were reduced after adequate therapy. Eleven of these patients also had symptoms of urethritis. The 7 patients with Chlamydia were all cured of their infection. These 7 patients had symptoms of prostatitis (rectal palpation disclosed a swollen, painful prostate), as well as urethritis. *C. trachomatis* was isolated from the

Table 5. Frequency of isolations of Mycoplasma, Ureaplasma or Chlamydia alone and of combinations of these agents from patients with "non-specific" prostatitis and effect of anti-microbial therapy.

Organisms isolated	No. of patients (n = 85)	No. of patients free of symptoms after therapy
Mycoplasma hominis	2	0
Ureaplasma urealyticum	30	10
M. hominis + U. urealyticum	8	2
Chlamydia trachomatis	5	5
C. trachomatis + U. urealyticum	2	2
Only "commensal" flora	38*	3

* Only 18 were treated in the same way as the other patients (see text).

Table 6. Isolation of various serotypes of *U. urealyticum* from patients with "non-specific" prostatitis and from healthy controls.

Serotype	No. of patients	No. of healthy controls
1	6 (4)*	4
2	3 (2)	1
3	9 (3)	1
4	2 (2)	2
5	0	0
6	10	3
7	2	0
8	4	1
9?	0	1
7 + 4	1 (1)	0
unknown	1	0
Total	38 (12)	13

* Number of patients who became free of symptoms after eradication of Ureaplasma with tetracycline.

urethral sample from all 7 patients. Eighteen of the 38 patients from whom only commensal flora could be cultured were treated in the same way. Three became free of complaints. The other 20 patients were treated with tetracycline during 25 days alone or had tetracycline therapy in the past without success.

All strains of *U. urealyticum* were serotyped by means of indirect immunofluorescence. The results are shown in Table 6. One strain was lost and could not be serotyped. One strain was initially serotyped as serotype 9 but further study created doubts. The strain is still studied at the moment.

Discussion

Approximately 15% of the patients with clinically diagnosed chronic prostatitis had chronic prostatitis due to bacteria. Anaerobic bacteria seem to be of minor importance in prostatitis. They may possibly play a role in prostatic abscesses, from which they have been isolated in significant numbers (FISHBACH and FINEGOLD, 1973; BARTLETT et al., 1978). From the results of our study it cannot be concluded that there is any relationship between viruses and chronic prostatitis. The results of similar virological studies (NIELSEN and VESTERGAARD, 1973; MÅRDH and COLLEEN, 1975) are in conformity with our results.

Trichomonas vaginalis and yeasts seem to be the cause of chronic prostatitis in only a small percentage of all cases. *M. hominis* probably doesn't play any role in the pathogenesis of chronic prostatitis.

The difference in frequency of isolation of *U. urealyticum* between patients with "non-specific" prostatitis (prostatitis not caused by known urogenital pathogens) and healthy controls was significant. However from this cannot be concluded that there is an aetiological relationship between *U. urealyticum* and chronic "non-specific" prostatitis. It is possible that the patients with prostatitis had more sexual partners than the control group but we have no data with which to evaluate this possibility. It is well known that the rate of colonization with Ureaplasma is closely associated with the number of sexual partners (McCORMACK et al., 1973).

After treatment with tetracycline or doxycycline all ureaplasmas were eradicated and about one-third of the patients became free of symptoms. Besides the fact that these 12 patients who became free of symptoms, had high leucocyte counts in their prostatic fluid, eleven of them also had symptoms of urethritis. All isolated strains of Ureaplasma were serotyped. The figures were too small for statistical analysis and allowed tentative conclusions only. It appeared that there was no distinct difference in the distribution of serotypes of Ureaplasma between patients and healthy men. Furthermore, no relation could be demonstrated between a favourable outcome of tetracycline therapy and particular serotypes.

Although from several patients with prostatitis *C. trachomatis* was isolated from prostatic fluid, urine after prostatic massage and seminal fluid these patients also had symptoms of urethritis. The organism was isolated in all cases from the urethral samples.

The results of this study suggest that *Ureaplasma urealyticum* plays a role in the pathogenesis of certain cases of prostatitis and also suggest that *Chlamydia trachomatis* urethritis can extend to the prostate gland. Urethritis accompanying the prostatitis seems to indicate a favourable prognosis. Furthermore, it is our opinion, that in patients with clinical symptoms of chronic prostatitis, who have no leucocytes in urine, prostatic fluid or seminal fluid, extensive microbiological studies are not indicated. In these cases, infection is not the cause of the patient's condition.

References

(1) BARTLETT, J. G., W. M. WEINSTEIN, S. L. GORBACH: Prostatic abscesses involving anaerobic bacteria. Arch. intern. Med. *138*: 1369 (1978).

(2) BLACK, F. T., A. KROGSGAARD-JENSEN: Application of indirect immunofluorescence, indirect haemagglutination and polyacrylamide-gel electrophoresis to human T-mycoplasmas. Acta path. microbiol. scand. Section B. *82*: 345 (1974).

(3) CROY, T. R., C.-C. KUO, S.-P. WANG: Comparative susceptibility of eleven mammalian cell lines to infection with trachoma organisms. J. clin. Microbiol. *1*: 434 (1975).

(4) FISHBACH, R. S., S. M. FINEGOLD: Anaerobic prostatic abscess with bacteremia. Amer. J. clin. Path. *59*: 408 (1973).

(5) HERDERSCHEÊ, D.: An improved medium for the cultivation of the Eaton agent. Antonie van Leeuwenhoek *29*: 154 (1963).

(6) KUO, C.-C., S.-P. WANG, J. T. GRAYSTON: Growth of trachoma organisms in HeLa 229 cell culture. In: HOBSON, D., K. K. HOLMES (eds.): Nongonococcal urethritis and related infections; p. 328. American Society for Microbiology, Washington, D.C. 1977.

(7) LASH, J. J.: A simplified casein hydrolisate-serum medium for the cultivation of *Trichomonas vaginalis*. Amer. J. trop. Med. *30*: 641 (1950).

(8) LENNETTE, E. H., N. J. SCHMIDT: Diagnostic procedures for viral and rickettsial infections, 4th edition. American Public Health Association, New York 1969.

(9) MÅRDH, P.-A., S. COLLEEN: Search for uro-genital tract infections in patients with symptoms of prostatitis. Scand. J. Urol. Nephrol. *9*: 8 (1975).

(10) McCORMACK, W. M., Y.-H. LEE, S. H. ZINNER: Sexual experience and urethral colonization with genital mycoplasmas. A study in normal men. Ann. intern. Med. *78*: 696 (1973).

(11) NIELSEN, M. L., B. F. VESTERGAARD: Virological investigations in chronic prostatitis. J. Urol. (Baltimore) *109*: 1023 (1973).

(12) PANANGALA, V. S., D. H. LEIN: Development of a template for use in immunofluorescent identification of mycoplasmas. J. clin. Microbiol. *7*: 399 (1978).

(13) SHEPARD, M. C., C. D. LUNCEFORD: Urease color test medium U-9 for the detection and identification of „T" mycoplasmas in clinical material. Appl. Microbiol. *20*: 539 (1970).

(14) SHEPARD, M. C., C. D. LUNCEFORD: Differential agar medium (A7) for identification of *Ureaplasma urealyticum* (human T mycoplasmas) in primary cultures of clinical material. J. clin. Microbiol. *3*: 613 (1976).

(15) SHEPARD, M. C., C. D. LUNCEFORD: Serological typing of Ureaplasma urealyticum isolates from urethritis patients by an agar growth inhibition method. J. clin. Microbiol. *8*, 566 (1978).

(16) THAYER, J. D., J. E. MARTIN jr.: Improved medium selective for cultivation of N. gonorrhoeae and N. meningitidis. Publ. Hlth. Reg. *81*: 559 (1966).

(17) WANG, S.-P., J. T. GRAYSTON: Human serology in Chlamydia trachomatis infection with microimmunofluorescence. J. infect. Dis. *130*: 388 (1974).

Institut für Medizinische Mikrobiologie und Virologie der Universität Düsseldorf;
Abteilung für Urologie; Institut für Medizinische Mikrobiologie der Universität Gießen

Studies on the Role of Ureaplasma urealyticum and Mycoplasma hominis in Prostatitis*

H. BRUNNER, W. WEIDNER, H. G. SCHIEFER

Abstract

It has definitely been demonstrated that *Ureaplasma urealyticum* is one etiologic agent of nongonococcal urethritis, a sexually transmitted disease. For this reason it seemed possible that the organisms might cause ascending inflammatory reactions of the prostate. Quantitative determinations of ureaplasmas and *Mycoplasma hominis,* together with localization studies, were therefore performed to elucidate the importance of these microorganisms in patients with chronic prostatitis. *U. urealyticum* was found in high numbers in expressed prostatic secretions and urine voided after prostatic massage from 82 (13.7%) of 597 patients with chronic prostatitis. Because numbers of ureaplasmas in first-voided urine and midstream urine were significantly lower, the source of the organisms in these patients was assumed to be the prostate. These data and the results of tetracycline treatment provide sufficient evidence for the etiologic importance of ureaplasmas in chronic prostatitis.

Introduction

Chlamydia trachomatis is the most important etiologic agent of nongonococcal urethritis, accounting for ~50% of cases (1). In addition, conclusive evidence indicates that *Ureaplasma urealyticum* plays a causative role in some men with nongonococcal urethritis (2). Support for the etiologic role of *U. urealyticum* in nongonococcal urethritis has been provided by qualitative and quantitative isolation studies and studies of the response to antibiotic therapy in humans and by intraurethral inoculation of chimpanzees (2−9). Recently, TAYLOR-ROBINSON et al. succeeded in fulfilling Koch's postulates by intraurethral

---

* This paper is originally published in *"The Journal of Infectious Diseases" 147*: 807−813 (1983), and is printed by permission of the University of Chicago Press, Chicago, Ill.

inoculation of ureaplasmas in men, causing relatively severe disease symptoms (10). On the other hand, a definite statement about the frequency in which these microorganisms act as primary pathogens in nongonococcal urethritis cannot be made at the present time.

Because ureaplasmas and *Mycoplasma hominis* can be found in the urethras of a high percentage of healthy men, the mere isolation of these organisms from the urethra cannot be considered to indicate that they are the etiologic agents of genital tract disease in an individual patient (11, 12). *M. hominis* has been demonstrated to cause upper urinary tract infections, but using quantitative culture procedures, these microorganisms could not be associated with nongonococcal urethritis (3, 13).

Because the etiology and the pathogenesis of chronic prostatitis are poorly understood at the present time, a study was started in 1975 in which, besides common bacteria, *U. urealyticum* and *M. hominis* were cultured quantitatively from patients with prostatitis. For localization of the infection, the four-specimen technique described by MEARES and STAMEY was used, and the response of symptoms to tetracycline therapy was compared with microbiologic findings after treatment (14). Patients from whom *Neisseria gonorrhoeae* or *C. trachomatis* could be isolated were excluded from the study.

Materials and methods

Patients: During the period of 1975–1980, a total of 597 men (mean age, 41 years) attended the special prostatitis outpatient clinic. Typically, patients with prostatitis complained of variable symptoms, such as urinary frequency, urgency, nocturia, terminal dysuria, abdominal aching, backache, or testicular, penile, or perineal pain. Some men were asymptomatic. In these cases prostatic tenderness or edema at rectal examination was the reason for further diagnostic procedures. A full medical history was taken for all patients.

Patients with urethral discharge (urethritis) and upper urinary tract infection by common bacteria were not included in the study. Men who had taken antibiotics within four weeks before attendance were excluded. The patients were categorized according to the following criteria.

Thirty-two of the 597 patients (mean age, 41 years) had chronic bacterial prostatitis. In the four-specimen technique of MEARES and STAMEY (14), $>10^4$ cfu of gram-negative rods per milliliter of fluid (24 men, 19 with *Escherichia coli*) or of *Streptococcus faecalis* (8 men) were isolated from expressed prostatic secretions (EPS) and $>10^3$ cfu per milliliter of fluid from urine voided after prostatic massage (VB3). In all of these patients, first voided urine (VB1) and midstream urine (VB2) contained at least 10-fold lower numbers of bacteria, indicating that the organisms were localized predominantly in the prostate (14). Furthermore, leukocyturia of ≥ 5, using a magnification of 400, was seen in the sediment of VB3 (15).

In 187 patients (mean age, 39 years) prostatodynia was the diagnosis. All patients with infections caused by Enterobacteriaceae, enterococci, and ureaplasmas as etiologic agents were excluded using the quantitative criteria mentioned above.

Furthermore, the sediment of VB3 contained less than five leukocytes per milliliter. All patients with infections caused by *N. gonorrhoeae,* urethral commensals in high numbers (for example, *Staphylococcus aureus* and group B *Streptococcus*), *Trichomonas vaginalis,* and *Candida* species were excluded.

Ureaplasma-associated prostatitis was defined by the presence of $\geq 10^4$ cfu of *U. urealyticum*/ml of EPS and, in the majority of cases, also by detection of $> 10^3$ cfu of *U. urealyticum*/ml of VB3. In these patients VB1 and VB2 contained at least 10-fold lower numbers of ureaplasmas than EPS or VB3. Because of lack of knowledge of the cellular inflammatory reaction during mycoplasmal disease, the leukocyte count, according to DRACH and KOHNEN (15), was not regarded as essential for this group of patients. In these men one negative culture for *C. trachomatis* of a urethral swab after prostatic massage was required.

Furthermore, 48 healthy volunteers (mean age, 42.5 years) were studied.

Sampling: In all men, VB1, VB2, EPS, and VB3 (~ 10 ml) were obtained, as described by MEARES and STAMEY (14). The localization studies were performed as shown in Table 1. In addition, blood was taken for syphilis serology, and uroflowmetric studies were performed to exclude patients with obstructive disorders of the urinary tract.

Table 1. Localization studies of infectious agents in men with prostatitis.

Term	Definition	Studies
VB1	First voided urine	Quantitative determination of common bacteria, mycoplasmas, and fungi
VB2	Midstream urine	As for VB1; number of leukocytes in sediment
EPS	Expressed prostatic secretions	As for VB1; cultured for *Neisseria gonorrhoeae* and *Chlamydia trachomatis**
VB3	Urine voided after prostatic massage	As for VB1; microscopy and culture for *Trichomonas vaginalis;* number of leukocytes in sediment

* It was not possible to determine routinely the number of leukocytes in EPS because all available material was used for the microbiologic tests.

Handling of specimens: For presence of mycoplasmas, urine specimens were cultured not later than 3 hr after collection. EPS (0.01 ml), taken from the meatus urethrae with a calibrated bacteriologic loop, was transferred to 2 ml of a fluid transport medium, designed to preserve ureaplasmas for at least 72 hr at room temperature (about 20 C) without permitting growth of the organisms, even when the medium was exposed to 37 C. Subsequently, 0.1 ml of each urine specimen and 0.1 ml of the transport medium were inoculated on A6-D agar, described by SHEPARD (16), and on a standard mycoplasmal agar (17). In addition, two broths (U-9 and standard broth) were inoculated with 0.1 ml of the transport medium containing EPS and 0.1 ml of urine sediment after centrifugation of ~10 ml of urine for 10 min at 1,000 g (17, 18).

Tests for bacterial, fungal, or trichomonadal infections were performed by standard techniques. The number of common bacteria and *Candida* species was determined semiquantitatively using calibrated bacteriologic loops (19, 20). EPS was examined for the presence of gonococci by Gram stain and culture on Thayer-Martin medium. In addition, the presence of *T. vaginalis* was determined microscopically and by culture procedures (21). Infections with bacteria other than ureaplasmas and with chlamydiae, fungi, or *T. vaginalis* are not described in detail in this report. An endourethral specimen was taken for isolation of *C. trachomatis* on cycloheximide-treated McCoy cells (22).

Media: The transport medium consisted of PPLO broth (Difco Laboratories, Detroit) supplemented with 1% PPLO serum fraction (Difco). HAYFLICK's formula was used for the standard mycoplasmal agar and broth (17, 23). The agar medium A6-D and the fluid medium U-9 for the cultivation of ureaplasmas were used, as described by SHEPARD (16) and SHEPARD and LUNCEFORD (18). Because it was later reported (24) that the level of manganese salt in A6-D agar was somewhat inhibitory to certain serotypes of *U. urealyticum,* we recommend the use of A7-B differential agar for subsequent similar studies.

Cultivation procedures: Agar plates inoculated with the four specimens of each patient were incubated for five days at 37 C, using the Gas Pak System (BBL, Heidelberg). Colonies were then counted using a dissecting microscope at a magnification of 25, and the number of cfu present in the original specimen was calculated. The fluid media, incubated at 37 C for five days, were inspected twice daily for a color change of the phenol red indicator. When a shift to the alkaline reaction occurred without turbidity, a subculture was made on the agar media described above. It was of utmost importance to perform the subculturing as early as possible; because a strong alkaline shift of the medium was toxic for ureaplasmas, subculture could be unsuccessful, whereas the original agar media showed growth of the organisms.

Identification of isolates: U. urealyticum was identified by its typical colony morphology, the ability to produce urease, and its resistance to lincomycin. *M.*

hominis and *Mycoplasma fermentans* were identified by epifluorescence using specific antisera to the organisms (25).

Treatment: Patients with *Ureaplasma*-associated prostatitis received 500 mg of tetracycline hydrochloride twice a day for 14 days. They were re-examined and samples were collected again 21−28 days after the start of treatment, using the quantitative techniques described above.

Statistical analysis: Statistical analyses were performed as described by CLAUSS and EBNER (26).

Results

Isolation and quantitative determination of U. urealyticum in patients with prostatitis: *U. urealyticum* could be isolated from various specimens of 6.0%−20.3% of the 597 men with prostatitis (Table 2). The highest isolation rate (20.3%) was found in EPS. More than 10^3 cfu of *U. urealyticum*/ml was found in VB1 of 14 of 70 men, in VB2 of nine of 36 men, in EPS of 93 of 121

Table 2. Isolation, quantitative determination, and localization of *Ureaplasma urealyticum* in 597 men with chronic prostatitis.

Specimen*	*U. urealyticum* (cfu/ml)	Isolation	Constellation Prostatitis** A	B	C	Prostatourethritis
VB1	$<10^3$ $>10^3$	56 14 } 70 (11.7%)	18 0	0 0	0 2	0 12
VB2	$<10^3$ $>10^3$	27 9 } 36 (6.0%)	12 0	0 0	1 1	0 8
EPS	$<10^3$ 10^3-10^4 $>10^4$	28 36 57*** } 121 (20.3%)	0 27 22	0 0 31	0 0 2	0 9 0
VB3	$<10^3$ $>10^3$	42 52**** } 94 (15.7%)	0 49	31 0	0 2	0 0

   * Localization of the infection (14): prostate, highest number of organisms in expressed prostatic secretions (EPS) and urine voided after prostatic massage (VB3); urethra, highest number of organisms in first voided urine (VB1); and upper urinary tract, highest number of organisms in midstream urine (VB2).

  ** Groups A (49 men), B (31 men), and C (2 men) represent patients with *Ureaplasma*-associated prostatitis but with a different distribution of organisms among the four specimens.

 *** Two patients also had high numbers of *Escherichia coli.*

**** One patient also had high numbers of *E. coli.*

men, and in VB3 of 52 of 94 men. The number of cfu in VB3 was significantly higher than in VB1 (U = 4.72, P < 0.01).

Prostatitis constellation for U. urealyticum: In 82 patients a typical prostatitis constellation for *U. urealyticum* was observed (Table 2). These patients could be assigned to three groups, designated A, B, and C. In 49 patients (group A), $>10^3$ cfu/ml was isolated from EPS and VB3 and $<10^3$ ureaplasmas/ml was found in VB1 and VB2. In 31 patients (group B), $>10^4$ cfu/ml was found in EPS, 600−1,000 cfu/ml in VB3, and no ureaplasmas in VB1 and VB2. In two men (group C), high numbers ($>10^3$ cfu/ml) in EPS and VB3 were accompanied by $>10^3$ cfu/ml in VB1 and VB2, but in both cases VB1 and VB2 contained at least 10-fold fewer organisms than EPS and VB3. In all three groups (total, 82 patients), the findings were in agreement with the definition of prostatitis by MEARES and STAMEY (14). These men were therefore considered to have *Ureaplasma*-associated prostatitis. Furthermore, three patients harbored high numbers of *U. urealyticum* in either EPS (two patients) or VB3 (one patient) and $<10^3$ cfu/ml of VB1 and VB2. In these three patients, a mixed infection with gram-negative rods *(E. coli)* was seen, and the prostatitis histogram could therefore not be associated with a single agent.

Prostato-urethritis constellation for U. urealyticum: Twelve patients had high numbers of ureaplasmas in VB1 (Table 2). In nine of these men, $>10^3$ cfu of *U. urealyticum*/ml was also observed in EPS. In these nine men, the infection could not be localized to either the urethra or the prostate and was therefore considered as prostato-urethritis.

Isolation and quantitative determination of M. hominis in patients with prostatitis: *M. hominis* was cultured from 2.8%−5.9% of various specimens from patients with prostatitis (Table 3). The highest isolation rate was seen in EPS. From 14 of 25 VB1 specimens and 11 of 17 VB2 samples, *M. hominis* was cultured in numbers of $>10^3$ cfu/ml. In contrast to isolation of *Ureaplasma,* in these cases no significant difference was seen in the isolation rate from EPS (28 of 35) and VB3 (six of 28).

Prostatitis constellation for M. hominis: A typical prostatitis histogram for *M. hominis* was evident in 10 patients (Table 3), but in all patients a mixed infection with high numbers of *U. urealyticum* (7 patients), *E. coli* (2 patients), or *S. faecalis* (1 patient) was observed. The prostatitis configuration could therefore not be assigned to *M. hominis* alone. In 11 additional patients, *M. hominis* could be isolated from VB1, VB2, and EPS in high numbers, but a prostatitis histogram was not seen.

Isolation and quantitative determination of U. urealyticum and M. hominis in healthy controls: In 8 (16.7%) of 48 healthy men ureaplasmas could also be isolated (Table 4). In contrast to patients with prostatitis, the highest isolation rate in this group was seen in VB1. In healthy men *U. urealyticum* was always

Table 3. Isolation, quantitative determination, and localization of *Mycoplasma hominis* in 597 patients with chronic prostatitis.

Specimen*	*M. hominis* (cfu/ml)	Isolation	Constellation	
			Prostatitis	Upper UTI**
VB1	$<10^3$	11 } 25 (4.2%)	0	0
	$>10^3$	14	0	12
VB2	$<10^3$	6 } 17 (2.8%)	0	1
	$>10^3$	11	0	11
EPS	$<10^3$	7	0	1
	10^3-10^4	11 } 35 (5.9%)	0	4
	$>10^4$	17	10***	7
VB3	$<10^3$	22 } 28 (4.7%)	0	0
	$>10^3$	6	3***	0

Note. No prostatitis configuration was seen for *M. hominis* as a single infectious agent.
   * Localization of the infection (14): prostate, highest number of organisms in expressed prostatic secretions (EPS) and urine voided after prostatic massage (VB3); urethra, highest number of organisms in first voided urine (VB1); and upper urinary tract, highest number of organisms in midstream urine (VB2).
  ** UTI = urinary tract infection.
*** Mixed infection with *Ureaplasma urealyticum* (7 patients), *Escherichia coli* (2 patients), or *Streptococcus faecalis* (1 patient).

Table 4. Isolation, quantitative determination, and localization of mycoplasmas in 48 healthy men.

Organisms isolated	VB1	VB2	EPS	VB3
Ureaplasma urealyticum	8 $(10^{1.6})$	0	3 $(10^{2.8})$	3 $(10^{2.0})$
Mycoplasma hominis	6 $(<10^{1.0})$	0	1 $(>10^{4.0})$	1 $(10^{3.7})$
Total	14	0	4	4

Note. Data are no. of men from whom mycoplasmas could be isolated (titer, in cfu/ml). VB1 = first voided urine; VB2 = midstream urine; EPS = expressed prostatic secretions; and VB3 = urine voided after prostatic massage.

isolated in numbers of $<10^3$ cfu/ml. *M. hominis* was detected in six additional men (12.5%), in all cases in VB1 and in only one case also in EPS and VB3. This man had high numbers of *M. hominis* in EPS ($>10^4$ cfu/ml) and VB3 ($10^{3.7}$ cfu/ml).

Therapy: The 82 patients with a typical *Ureaplasma*-associated prostatitis histogram were treated with 500 mg of tetracycline hydrochloride twice a day for 14 days. Seventy-one of these patients were free of symptoms and ureaplasmas could not be detected 21−28 days after the start of treatment. In the remaining 11 patients with persistent symptoms, seven had severe bladder neck obstruction, which might explain the unsuccessful results of treatment; in four patients failure of therapy was unexplained.

Discussion

Acute prostatitis due to a bacterial infection with a common urinary tract pathogen is a relatively rare event, and diagnostic difficulties are seldom encountered (27). On the other hand, chronic prostatitis is a common disease requiring rather elaborate diagnostic procedures, including quantitative evaluation of microorganisms in the four-specimen technique described by MEARES and STAMEY (14). Although this technique has been available for some time, the etiology of the disease is still poorly understood in >50% of patients with chronic prostatitis. Two very common forms of the disease have been distinguished: chronic bacterial prostatitis and nonbacterial prostatitis. Chronic bacterial prostatitis is caused by bacteria that are etiologic agents of acute prostatitis and other urogenital tract infections, whereas the etiology of chronic nonbacterial prostatitis is in most cases unknown. In addition, there is no clinical symptom pathognomonic for the disease (28−30). Therefore, quantitative microbiologic techniques and localization of the infection are of utmost importance for diagnosis and treatment of prostatitis.

As previously demonstrated (31) in patients with symptoms of prostatitis and a case history of more than two years, high numbers of *U. urealyticum* in EPS, VB3, and semen could be detected. In the present study, using the localization technique, 82 (13.7%) of 597 patients showed a typical histogram indicating *Ureaplasma*-associated prostatitis. Infections with other bacteria, including *C. trachomatis*, were not detected in these 82 men. In 9 additional patients from whom only *U. urealyticum* could be isolated in high numbers from EPS, an exact localization of the infection was not possible (see Table 2). These men also had high numbers of *U. urealyticum* in VB1 and VB2. This finding could indicate urethritis without spontaneous discharge or, more likely, prostato-urethritis. If these patients are included in the group with *Ureaplasma*-associated disease, the percentage of patients with prostatitis possibly caused by *U. urealyticum* is 15.2%. Quantitative determinations of mycoplasmas in VB1, VB2, EPS, and VB3 have to the best of our knowledge not been reported before by other investigators.

In 8 of 48 healthy men *U. urealyticum* was also isolated, but never in the typical prostatitis configuration. These findings are in agreement with previous results indicating that numbers of ureaplasmas in healthy persons do not exceed 10^3 cfu/ml of VB1 (3, 31). In contrast to our findings, BOWIE et al. (32) and VIARENGO et al. (33) demonstrated in some healthy persons $>10^3$ color-changing units of *U. urealyticum*/ml of VB1. The difference from our findings can be explained by the use of color-changing units in the quantitative isolation procedures of the other investigators as compared with cfu in our studies.

Based on our previous findings that patients with numbers of ureaplasmas of $<10^4$ cfu/ml of EPS and $<10^3$ cfu/ml of urine did not respond to tetracycline therapy whereas patients with higher numbers of ureaplasmas could be cured, only the 82 patients with a histogram of *Ureaplasma*-associated prostatitis were treated with tetracycline hydrochloride. In these experiments we could confirm previous results regarding successful tetracycline treatment (3). 71 of the 82 patients responded to this therapy. Failures of treatment and persistence of symptoms could be explained by bladder neck obstruction, reinfection via the sexual partner, or the presence of tetracycline-resistant ureaplasmas, as previously observed by other investigators (9, 34). It must be emphasized that, despite the fact that ureaplasmas could be cultivated again after therapy in some cases, a typical prostatitis histogram was not observed. Because a new species of *Mycoplasma* has recently been isolated from the human urethra, another tetracycline-sensitive microorganism must be discussed as an etiologic agent (35).

Leukocyte counts in EPS would be required to include patients with the *Ureaplasma*-associated prostatitis histogram in the bacterial prostatitis group, according to DRACH and KOHNEN (15) and DRACH (36). The determination of leukocyte numbers was not possible because all of the EPS available from the patients was needed for the microbiologic tests. In a separate group of patients, we were recently able to demonstrate higher numbers of polymorphonuclear leukocytes and macrophages in VB3 in *Ureaplasma*-associated prostatitis as compared with those in prostatodynia (authors' unpublished observations). We therefore suggest that patients with *Ureaplasma*-associated prostatitis be included in the bacterial prostatitis group.

The presented quantitative determinations of *U. urealyticum* in $\sim 14\% - 15\%$ of our patients with chronic prostatitis suggest, but do not prove, that these microorganisms are the etiologic agents of the disease in these patients. Further evidence could be provided by detection of specific local or serum antibodies to *U. urealyticum* and by eventually showing predominance of certain serotypes in patients with high numbers of ureaplasmas (30).

As far as diagnostic procedures in a patient with chronic prostatitis are concerned, our findings indicate that, similar to in a patient with nongonococcal urethritis, quantitative determinations of *U. urealyticum* should be performed. Isolation alone is clearly not sufficient for diagnostic purposes until sensitive serologic procedures for antibody detection are available or virulent organisms can be separated from commensals by other techniques.

As expected, mixed infections with *U. urealyticum* and gram-negative bacteria or enterococci were seen. Because patients with *C. trachomatis* were excluded, the simultaneous occurrence of *C. trachomatis* with high numbers of ureaplasmas cannot be discussed. *C. trachomatis* has been found in some patients with acute epididymitis and should be considered as a possible etiologic agent of chronic prostatitis (37). A typical prostatitis histogram for *M. hominis* was not found in our patient group but was found in one of the healthy men. These findings argue against *M. hominis* as an etiologic agent of prostatitis. On the other hand, *M. hominis* was found in high numbers in VB1 and VB2 in 11 of our patients. This finding supports previous results showing that *M. hominis* might cause upper urinary tract infections (13).

Acknowledgements

This research was supported by funds from the Deutsche Forschungsgemeinschaft, Bonn-Bad Godesberg.
We thank M. Ludwig and U. Gerhard for technical assistance.

References

(1) Taylor-Robinson, D., B. J. Thomas: The role of *Chlamydia trachomatis* in genital-tract and associated diseases. J. Clin. Pathol. *33*: 205−233 (1980).

(2) Taylor-Robinson, D., W. M. McCormack: The genital mycoplasmas (parts 1 and 2). N. Engl. J. Med. *302*: 1003−1010, 1063−1067 (1980).

(3) Weidner, W., H. Brunner, W. Krause, C. F. Rothauge: The importance of *Ureaplasma urealyticum* in non-specific prostato-urethritis. Dtsch. Med. Wochenschr. *103*: 465−470 (1978).

(4) Shepard, M. C.: Quantitative relationship of *Ureaplasma urealyticum* to the clinical course of nongonococcal urethritis in the human male. Institut National de la Santé et de la Recherche Médicale *33*: 375−379 (1974).

(5) Bowie, W. R., E. R. Alexander, J. F. Floyd, J. Holmes, Y. Miller, K. K. Holmes: Differential response of chlamydial and *Ureaplasma*-associated urethritis to sulphafurazole (sulfisoxazole) and aminocyclitols. Lancet *2*: 1276−1278 (1976).

(6) Coufalik, E. D., D. Taylor-Robinson, G. W. Csonka: Treatment of nongonococcal urethritis with rifampicin as a means of defining the role of *Ureaplasma urealyticum*. Br. J. Vener. Dis. *55*: 36−43 (1979).

(7) Munday, P. E., B. J. Thomas, A. P. Johnson, D. G. Altman, D. Taylor-Robinson: Clinical and microbiological study of nongonococcal urethritis with particular reference to non-chlamydial disease. Br. J. Vener. Dis. *57*: 327−333 (1981).

(8) Taylor-Robinson, D., R. H. Purcell, W. T. London, D. L. Sly: Urethral infection of chimpanzees by *Ureaplasma urealyticum*. J. Med. Microbiol. *11*: 197−201 (1978).

(9) Stimson, J. B., J. Hale, W. R. Bowie, K. K. Holmes: Tetracycline-resistant *Ureaplasma urealyticum:* a cause of persistent nongonococcal urethritis. Ann. Intern. Med. *94*: 192−194 (1981).

(10) TAYLOR-ROBINSON, D., G. W. CSONKA, M. J. PRENTICE: Human intra-urethral inoculation of ureaplasmas. Q. J. Med. *46*: 309−326 (1977).

(11) SHEPARD, M. C.: The recovery of pleuropneumonia-like organisms from Negro men with and without nongonococcal urethritis. American Journal of Syphilis, Gonorrhea, and Venereal Diseases *38*: 113−124 (1954).

(12) FOY, H., G. KENNY, E. BOR, S. HAMARR, R. HICKMAN: Prevalence of *Mycoplasma hominis* and *Ureaplasma urealyticum* (T strains) in urine of adolescents. J. Clin. Microbiol. *2*: 226−230 (1975).

(13) THOMSEN, A. C.: Occurrence of mycoplasmas in urinary tract of patients with acute pyelonephritis. J. Clin. Microbiol. *8*: 84−88 (1978).

(14) MEARES, E. M., T. A. STAMEY: Bacteriologic localization patterns in bacterial prostatitis and urethritis. Invest. Urol. *5*: 492−518 (1968).

(15) DRACH, G. W., P. KOHNEN: Prostatitis. In: TANNENBAUM, M. (ed.): Urologic pathology: the prostate; p. 157−170. Lea and Febiger, Philadelphia 1977.

(16) SHEPARD, M. C.: Differential methods for identification of T-mycoplasmas based on demonstration of urease. J. Infect. Dis. *127* (Suppl.): 22−25 (1973).

(17) CHANOCK, R. M., L. HAYFLICK, M. F. BARILE: Growth on artificial medium of an agent associated with atypical pneumonia and its identification as a PPLO. Proc. Natl. Acad. Sci. U.S.A. *48*: 41−49 (1962).

(18) SHEPARD, M. C., C. D. LUNCEFORD: Urease color test medium U-9 for the detection and identification of "T" mycoplasmas in clinical material. Applied Microbiology *20*: 539−543 (1970).

(19) KASS, E. H.: Bacteriuria and the diagnosis of infections of the urinary tract: a ten year gap. Arch. Intern. Med. *100*: 709−714 (1957).

(20) SILVA-HUTNER, M., B. H. COOPER: Yeasts of medical importance. In: LENNETTE, E. H., A. BALOWS, W. J. HAUSLER JR., J. P. TRUANT (eds.): Manual of clinical microbiology. 3rd ed.; p. 562−576. American Society for Microbiology, Washington, D.C. 1980.

(21) BROOKE, M. M., D. M. MELVIN: Intestinal and urogenital protozoa. In: LENNETTE, E. H., A. BALOWS, W. J. HAUSLER JR., J. P. TRUANT (eds.): Manual of clinical microbiology. 3rd ed.; p. 675−687. American Society for Microbiology, Washington, D.C. 1980.

(22) RIPA, K. T., P. A. MÅRDH: Cultivation of *Chlamydia trachomatis* in cycloheximide-treated McCoy cells. J. Clin. Microbiol. *6*: 328−331 (1977).

(23) HAYFLICK, L.: Tissue cultures and mycoplasmas. Tex. Rep. Biol. Med. *23* (Suppl. 1): 285−303 (1965).

(24) SHEPARD, M. C., R. S. COMBS: Enhancement of *Ureaplasma urealyticum* growth on a differential agar medium (A7B) by a polyamine, putrescine. J. Clin. Microbiol. *10*: 931−933 (1979).

(25) DELGIUDICE, R. A., N. F. ROBILLARD, T. R. CARSKI: Immunofluorescence identification of mycoplasma on agar by use of incident illumination. J. Bacteriol. *93*: 1205−1209 (1967).

(26) CLAUSS, G., H. EBNER: Grundlagen der Statistik. p. 250−251. Deutsch, Zürich 1975.

(27) MEARES, E. M., JR.: Bacterial prostatitis vs. "prostatosis" − a clinical and bacteriological study. J.A.M.A. *224*: 1372−1375 (1973).

(28) MOBLEY, D. F.: Chronic prostatitis. South. Med. J. *67*: 219−224 (1974).

(29) MEARES, E. M., JR.: Urinary tract infections in men. In: HARRISON J. H., R. F. GITTES, A. D. PERLMUTTER, T. A. STAMEY, P. C. WALSH (eds.): Campbell's urology. 4th ed.; p. 509−537. Saunders, Philadelphia 1979.

(30) MEARES, E. M., JR.: Serum antibody titers in urethritis and chronic bacterial prostatitis. Urology *10*: 305−309 (1977).

(31) WEIDNER, W., H. BRUNNER, W. KRAUSE: Quantitative culture of *Ureaplasma urealyticum* in patients with chronic prostatitis or prostatosis. J. Urol. *124*: 622−625 (1980).

(32) BOWIE, W. R., S. P. WANG, E. R. ALEXANDER, J. FLOYD, P. S. FORSYTH, H. M. POLLOCK, J. L. LIN, T. M. BUCHANAN, K. K. HOLMES: Etiology of nongonococcal urethritis: evidence for *Chlamydia trachomatis* and *Ureaplasma urealyticum*. J. Clin. Invest. *59*: 735−742 (1977).

(33) VIARENGO, J., F. HEBRANT, P. PIOT: *Ureaplasma urealyticum* in the urethra of healthy men. Br. J. Vener. Dis. *56*: 169−172 (1980).

(34) Evans, R. T., D. Taylor-Robinson: The incidence of tetracycline-resistant strains of *Ureaplasma urealyticum*. J. Antimicrob. Chemother. *4*: 57–63 (1978).

(35) Taylor-Robinson, D., J. G. Tully, P. M. Furr, R. M. Cole, D. L. Rose, N. F. Hanna: Urogenital mycoplasma infections of man: a review with observations on a recently discovered *Mycoplasma*. Isr. J. Med. Sci. *17*: 524–530 (1981).

(36) Drach, G. W.: Problems in diagnosis of bacterial prostatitis: gram-negative, gram-positive and mixed infections. J. Urol. *111*: 630–636 (1974).

(37) Berger, R. E., E. R. Alexander, J. P. Harnisch, C. A. Paulsen, G. D. Monda, J. Ansell, K. K. Holmes: Etiology, manifestations and therapy of acute epididymitis: prospective study of 50 cases. J. Urol. *121*: 750–754 (1979).

Institut für Medizinische Mikrobiologie; Urologische Universitätsklinik;
Institut für Hygiene und Infektionskrankheiten der Tiere, Abt. Zoonosen;
Dermatologische Universitätsklinik, Abt. Andrologie und Venerologie, der Universität Gießen

Prostatitis as Sequela of Non-Gonococcal Urethritis
A Prospective Study

H. G. Schiefer, W. Weidner, H. Krauss, U. Gerhardt, W. Krause

At present the etiology and pathogenesis of prostatitis are only partially understood (Meares, 1980). In case of acute and chronic prostatitis caused by common bacteria, the infected urine passing the prostatic section of the urethra, is assumed to convey enterobacteriae and enterococci into the prostate, mainly by reflux. In case of "abacterial" prostatitis, ureaplasmas and/or chlamydiae are hypothesized to be involved as etiologic agents. Both microorganisms are known to be the main pathogens causing non- and post-gonococcal urethritis (Cassell et al., 1981; Taylor-Robinson et al., 1980a, 1980b; Schachter, 1978; Weidner et al., 1980b, 1982). The assumption appears plausible that, by way of intracanalicular ascension, they might subsequently infect the prostate. Since this hypothesis has not yet been tested in a controlled clinical trial, we designed a prospective study of patients with non-gonococcal urethritis (NGU).

Patients and diagnostic procedures

Patients: 69 men (age, 20—50 years) suffering from acute non-gonococcal urethritis, attended the special prostatitis outpatient clinic (Prostatitis-Sprechstunde, Urologische Klinik, Justus-Liebig-Universität Gießen). The main clinical symptom was spontaneous urethral discharge combined with burning sensations when voiding. Patients with microscopically and/or culturally proved gonorrhoea, and patients with an anamnesis longer than four weeks were excluded from this study.

Microbiological studies: All microbiological investigations were done as previously described (Brunner et al., 1983; Weidner et al., 1978, 1980a, 1980b, 1982). All cultures were examined without knowledge of the clinical findings and diagnoses. Evaluation of data was done after completion of this study.

Diagnostics of urethritis: The diagnostic procedures and criteria for etiologic classification are listed in Table 1. The microbiological analysis of the urethral

Table 1. Diagnostic procedures and criteria for etiologic classification of *urethritis*.

1. Leading clinical symptom:	Urethral discharge
2. Microbiological analysis	
– urethral discharge:	Gram smear
	Common bacteria
	Neisseria gonorrhoeae
	Fungi
	Mycoplasmas
	Chlamydia trachomatis
– first voided urine (VB1):	Cytological analysis (PAPANICOLAOU)
	Common bacteria
	Fungi
	Mycoplasmas
	Trichomonas vaginalis

Etiologic classification is based on following criteria:
1. Isolation of Chlamydia trachomatis
2. Isolation of Neisseria gonorrhoeae
3. High numbers of Ureaplasma urealyticum
  i.e. $\geq 10^4$ cfu/ml urethral discharge
        $\geq 10^3$ cfu/ml first voided urine (VB1)
4. High numbers of common bacteria
  i.e. $\geq 10^4$ cfu/ml urethral discharge
        $\geq 10^3$ cfu/ml first voided urine (VB1)

discharge and the first voided urine specimens included the isolation and quantitative determination of common bacteria, fungi, and mycoplasmas, and the cultivation of Neisseria gonorrhoeae and Chlamydia trachomatis from the urethral discharge (WEIDNER et al., 1978, 1980a, 1980b, 1982).

Therapy: All patients with NGU were treated with 500 mg of tetracycline hydrochloride twice a day for two weeks. The patients were urged to abstain from sexual intercourse or, at least, to use a preservative. The female consorts were not controlled simultaneously and remained untreated.

Follow-up Examination: Four weeks after their first attendance to the outpatient clinic all patients underwent a standardized control procedure. In patients with persistent urethral discharge, the diagnostic procedures for NGU (Table 1) were repeated. In patients without discharge, a localization study according to the four-specimens-technique (MEARES et al., 1968) was performed. The diagnostic procedures and criteria for etiologic classification are detailed in Table 2. First voided urine (VB1), bladder urine (VB2), prostatic secretions (EPS) obtained by standardized prostatic massage (p.m.), and urine voided after p.m. (VB3), were quantitatively analyzed for common bacteria, fungi, and mycoplasmas. In addition, EPS was cultivated for Neisseria gonorrhoeae and Chlamydia trachomatis. VB3 was microscopically examined for Trichomonas vaginalis. VB2 and VB3 samples were examined for polymorphonuclear leucocytes (PML): 3 ml each of VB2 and VB3 were cytocentrifuged, and the sedimented material was transferred to a slide and stained according to Papanicolaou. In case of VB2 samples free of PML (≤ 2), the total number of PML in VB3 was determined in five areas using a 400 fold magnification: ≤ 2 PML per microscopic field were regarded as normal; ≤ 4 PML as borderline value; and >4 PML as pathognomonic for prostatitis (WEIDNER et al., 1983a).

The etiologic classification of prostatitis was based on the microbiological results according to the criteria detailed in Table 2.

Table 2. Diagnostic procedures and criteria for etiologic classification of *prostatitis*.

Localization study according to MEARES and STAMEY
Microbiological analysis
  − first voided urine (VB1): Common bacteria
                              Fungi
                              Mycoplasmas
  − bladder urine (VB2):   Cytological analysis (PAPANICOLAOU)
                              Common bacteria
                              Fungi
                              Mycoplasmas
Standardized prostatic massage
(p.m.)
  − prostatic fluid (EPS)/
    urethral swab after p.m.: Common bacteria
                              Neisseria gonorrhoeae
                              Fungi
                              Mycoplasmas
                              Chlamydia trachomatis
  − urine voided after p.m.
    (VB3):   Cytological analysis (PAPANICOLAOU)
                              Common bacteria
                              Fungi
                              Mycoplasmas
                              Trichomonas vaginalis

Prostatitis is diagnosed when, in the sediment of 3 ml of VB3, >4 PML are seen per microscopic field at 400fold magnification.

Etiologic classification is based on following criteria:
1. Isolation of Chlamydia trachomatis from EPS/urethral swab after p.m.
2. Isolation of Neisseria gonorrhoeae from EPS/urethral swab after p.m.
3. High numbers of Ureaplasma urealyticum in prostatitis constellation
   i.e. $\geq 10^4$ cfu/ml EPS
        $\geq 10^3$ cfu/ml VB3
        $< 10^3$ cfu/ml VB1 and VB2
4. High numbers of common bacteria in prostatitis constellation
   i.e. $\geq 10^4$ cfu/ml EPS
        $\geq 10^3$ cfu/ml VB3
        $< 10^3$ cfu/ml VB1 and VB2

Urinary tract infection was diagnosed if all urine specimens contained $>10^5$ cfu of common bacteria per ml.

Epididymitis was clinically diagnosed from the painfully infiltrated, swollen epididymis.

Therapeutic results were evaluated by clinical and microbiological criteria. Clinical success was stated when the patient did not complain of any discomfort. According to microbiological criteria a therapeutic success was reported when the original pathogen had been eradicated. Patients with enduring urethritis, epididymitis, or prostatitis were considered therapeutic failures.

Results

69 patients with NGU were included in this prospective study. NGU was classified (see Table 1) according to the isolated microorganisms: 31 (44.9%) patients were infected with Chlamydia trachomatis (C+), 22 patients (31.9%) with Ureaplasma urealyticum (U+), 8 patients (11.6%) with both Chlamydia trachomatis + Ureaplasma urealyticum (C+, U+), and 8 patients (11.6%) with common bacteria (B+), i.e. enterococci and group B streptococci.

All patients with NGU received antibiotic treatment. Four weeks after their first attendance all patients were re-examined, and samples were analyzed.

Following Chlamydia trachomatis-positive NGU (C+) (Table 3), clinical cure after tetracycline treatment occurred in 15 of 31 patients although chlamy-

Table 3. Prostatitis following NGU (C+) (n = 31).

Therapeutic result	Clincal symptoms	n	C+	U+	Other bacteria	Leucocytes	Classification of urogenital infection
Success	No symptoms	15					
		15	4	–	–	–	–
		16					
Failure	Urethral discharge	3	2	–	1 (GO)	3	Urethritis
	Symptoms of epididymitis	1	1	–	–	1	Epididymitis
	Symptoms of prostatitis	12	9	–	–	12	Prostatitis

diae could still be isolated from the urethra of 4 men after prostatic massage. Three patients continuously suffered from urethritis, two of them were still infected with chlamydiae, and from the urethral discharge of one patient gonococci could now be grown. Chlamydia-positive epididymitis developed in 1 man. Prostatitis, as indicated by high numbers of PML in urine after prostatic massage (VB3), had developed in 12 patients. From the prostatic fluids of 9 men C. trachomatis was cultivated.

Following Ureaplasma urealyticum-positive NGU (U+) (Table 4), clinical and microbiological cure after tetracycline treatment occurred in 16 of 22 patients. Therapy failed in 6 men: Urethritis persisted in 2 men. Prostatitis developed in 4 patients: in 2 of them ureaplasmas were cultivated in significantly high numbers from the prostatic fluid.

Following Chlamydia trachomatis- and Ureaplasma urealyticum-positive NGU (C+, U+) (Table 5), clinical cure after tetracycline treatment occurred in 4 of 8 patients, although chlamydiae could still be isolated from the urethra of 2 men. Therapy failed in 4 patients: in one man a chlamydia-positive gonococcal urethritis was diagnosed. Prostatitis developed in 2 patients. From the prostatic fluids of both patients C. trachomatis, and additionally in one case U. urealyticum, were cultivated.

Following bacterial NGU (B+) (Table 6), clinical cure after tetracycline treatment occurred in 4 of 8 patients. Therapy failed in 4 cases: two men continuously suffered from bacterial urethritis, and 2 men from urinary tract infection. In no case a prostatitis had developed.

Table 4. Prostatitis following NGU (U+) (n = 22).

Therapeutic result	Clinical symptoms	n	C+	U+	Other bacteria	Leucocytes	Classification of urogenital infection
Success	No symptoms	16					
		16	–	–	–	–	–
		6					
	Urethral discharge	2	1	1	–	2	Urethritis
Failure	Symptoms of epididymitis	–	–	–	–	–	–
	Symptoms of prostatitis	4	–	2	–	4	Prostatitis

Table 5. Prostatitis following NGU (C+, U+) (n = 8).

Therapeutic result	Clinical symptoms	n	C+	U+	Other bacteria	Leucocytes	Classification of urogenital infection
Success	No symptoms	4					
		4	2	–	–	–	–
		4					
Failure	Urethral discharge	1	1	–	1 (GO)	1	Urethritis
	Symptoms of epididymitis	1	1	–	–	–	Epididymitis
	Symptoms of prostatitis	2	2	1	–	2	Prostatitis

Table 6. Prostatitis following NGU (B+) (n = 8).

Therapeutic result	Clinical symptoms	n	C+	U+	Other bacteria	Leucocytes	Classification of urogenital infection
Success	No symptoms	4					
		4	–	–	–	–	–
		4					
Failure	Urethral discharge	2	–	–	2	2	Urethritis
	Symptoms of epididymitis	–	–	–	–	–	–
	Symptoms of prostatitis	–	–	–	–	–	–
	Urinary tract infection	2	–	–	2	2	Urinary tract infection

Discussion

Whereas the etiologic significance of Ureaplasma urealyticum and Chlamydia trachomatis for the pathogenesis of NGU is now well established (CASSELL et al., 1981; TAYLOR-ROBINSON et al., 1980; WEIDNER et al., 1980b, 1982), their role in prostatitis is still debatable.

The main difficulties in interpreting isolation experiments and results, arise from the fact that the prostatic secretions have to pass the urethra, and therefore the cultivated microorganisms might have originated from the urethral flora.

Regarding Ureaplasma urealyticum, we have demonstrated in recently published studies (BRUNNER et al., 1983; WEIDNER et al., 1980a) which included quantitative determinations of ureaplasmas and Mycoplasma hominis together with localization studies following the four-specimens-technique (MEARES et al., 1968), that U. urealyticum was isolated in significantly high numbers from the expressed prostatic secretions and urine voided after prostatic massage from 82 (13.7%) of 597 patients suffering from chronic prostatitis. The source of U. urealyticum in these patients was traced to be the prostate.

Regarding Chlamydia trachomatis, the data published in the literature, are highly controversial. MÅRDH et al. (1972) detected serum complement fixing antibody titers of $\geq$ 1:5 against chlamydiae in 33% of 79 men with non-acute prostatitis, compared to 3% of 72 blood donors as controls. The same authors (MÅRDH et al., 1978) published contradicting results: from 53 patients with chronic prostatitis (duration of symptoms, 6 months to 18 years) C. trachomatis was isolated from the urethral secretions of only one man, whereas from the prostatic secretions chlamydiae could not be grown. Serological evidence for C. trachomatis infections was also reported in only a few patients. Contrary to these negative results, JOHANNISSON (1981) and NILSSON et al. (1981) frequently isolated C. trachomatis from prostatic secretions of patients with subacute prostatitis. In previous studies (KRAUSS et al., 1983; WEIDNER et al., 1983b) we had obtained evidence that in cases of prostatitis a good correlation exists between cultivation of C. trachomatis as sole pathogen, high numbers of PML in VB3, and detection of humoral antibodies against C. trachomatis.

In the present prospective study, 69 patients with NGU were examined for the development of prostatitis. After initial diagnostic procedures all patients were treated with tetracycline since a longer lasting observation of untreated patients was considered unethical. All patients were re-examined four weeks after their first attendance to the clinic. Prostatitis was diagnosed when more than 4 PML were seen per microscopic field at 400 fold magnification in the sediment of 3 ml of urine voided after prostatic massage (VB 3) (WEIDNER et al., 1983a).

Prostatitis as sequela of NGU was observed in 18 (26%) of 69 patients, especially in those patients who had suffered from C. trachomatis-positive NGU. Furthermore an unexpectedly high rate of enduring chlamydial infections was detected.

For explanation some comments seem warranted.

In order to meet the objection that the cultivated chlamydiae might have originated from the urethra, we refer to the above mentioned correlation (KRAUSS et al., 1983; WEIDNER et al., 1983a) between isolation of C. trachomatis as sole pathogen in cases of prostatitis, high numbers of PML in VB3, and antibody response against C. trachomatis. In these cases C. trachomatis is considered the etiologic agent involved.

Concerning the high rate of enduring chlamydial infections despite tetracycline therapy, one must take into account several possibilities:

1. The compliance of our patients is unknown.
2. Persistent chlamydial infection may be due to the poor penetration of tetracycline into the prostate (MEARES, 1980).
3. Re-infection by the sexual consorts of our patients cannot be excluded since the females remained untreated.
4. Persistence is a common progression of the natural history of chlamydial infections (STORZ et al., 1977).

Frequently chlamydial infections are latent, and diseases chronical. Life-long infections despite antibiotic therapy have been observed. Persistence may be caused by the characteristic cell biology of chlamydiae. These microorganisms are obligate intracellular pathogens with a unique developmental life cycle (STORZ et al., 1977). Elementary bodies which are infectious, extracellular, metabolically inert, sporelike particles with a rigid cell wall enter into the cytoplasm of a host cell where they differentiate into vegetative, metabolically active, non-infectious reticulate bodies which finally form a new progeny of infectious elementary bodies prone to re-initiate the cycle of infection. These complex developmental processes occur only within endocytotic vesicles of the host cells into which most antibiotics can hardly penetrate so that therapy fails.

The existence of cryptic intracellular chlamydial forms and their significance for latency and persistence of chlamydial infections have been postulated (MOULDER et al., 1980).

Acknowledgement

The secretarial assistance of Agnes KRÖNER is gratefully acknowledged.

References

(1) BRUNNER, H., W. WEIDNER, H. G. SCHIEFER: Studies on the role of Ureaplasma urealyticum and Mycoplasma hominis in prostatitis. J. Infect. Diseas. *147*: 807−813 (1983).

(2) CASSELL, G. H., B. C. COLE: Mycoplasmas as agents of human disease. New Engl. J. Med. *304*: 80−89 (1981).

(3) JOHANNISSON, G.: Studies on Chlamydia trachomatis as a cause of lower urogenital tract infection. Acta Dermato-Venereologica (Stockholm) (Suppl.) *93* (1981).

(4) KRAUSS, H., H. G. SCHIEFER, W. WEIDNER, M. ARENS, H. EBNER: Significance of Chlamydia trachomatis in "abacterial" prostatitis. Zbl. Bakt. A *254*: 545−551 (1983).

(5) MÅRDH, P.-A., S. COLLEEN, B. HOLMQUIST: Chlamydia in chronic prostatitis. Brit. Med. J. *IV*: 361 (1972).

(6) MÅRDH, P.-A., K. T. RIPA, S. COLLEEN, J. D. TREHARNE, S. DAROUGAR: Role of Chlamydia trachomatis in non-acute prostatitis. Brit. J. Vener. Dis. *54*: 330−334 (1978).

(7) MEARES, E. M.: Prostatitis syndromes: new perspectives about old woes. J. Urol. *123*: 141−147 (1980).

(8) MEARES, E. M., T. A. STAMEY: Bacteriologic localization patterns in bacterial prostatitis and urethritis. Invest. Urol. *5*: 492−518 (1968).

(9) MOULDER, J. W., N. J. LEVY, L. P. SCHULMAN: Persistent infection of mouse fibroblasts (L cells) with Chlamydia psittaci: evidence for a cryptic chlamydial form. Infect. Immun. *30*: 874−883 (1980).

(10) NILSSON, S., G. JOHANNISSON, E. LYCKE: Isolation of Chlamydia trachomatis from the urethra and from prostatic fluid in men with signs and symptoms of acute urethritis. Acta Dermato-Venereologica *61*: 456−459 (1981).

(11) SCHACHTER, J.: Chlamydial infections. New Engl. J. Med. *298*: 428−435; 490−495; 540−549 (1978).

(12) STORZ, J., P. SPEARS: Chlamydiales: properties, cycle of development and effect on eukaryotic host cells. Curr. Top. Microbiol. Immunol. *76*: 167−214 (1977).

(13) TAYLOR-ROBINSON, D., W. M. McCORMACK: The genital mycoplasmas. New Engl. J. Med. *302*: 1003−1010; 1063−1067 (1980a).

(14) TAYLOR-ROBINSON, D., B. J. THOMAS: The rôle of Chlamydia trachomatis in genital-tract and associated diseases. J. Clin. Pathol. *33*: 205−233 (1980b).

(15) WEIDNER, W., H. BRUNNER, W. KRAUSE, C. F. ROTHAUGE: Zur Bedeutung von Ureaplasma urealyticum bei unspezifischer Prostato-Urethritis. Dtsch. Med. Wschr. *103*: 465−470 (1978).

(16) WEIDNER, W., H. BRUNNER, W. KRAUSE: Quantitative culture of Ureaplasma urealyticum in patients with chronic prostatitis or prostatosis. J. Urol. *124*: 622−625 (1980a).

(17) WEIDNER, W., H. G. SCHIEFER, H. KRAUSS, J. ENGSTFELD: Chlamydia trachomatis und Ureaplasma urealyticum bei unspezifischer Urethritis. Helv. chir. Acta *47*: 417−421 (1980b).

(18) WEIDNER, W., H. G. SCHIEFER, H. KRAUSS, J. ENGSTFELD: Untersuchungen zur Ätiologie der nicht-gonorrhoischen Urethritis. Dtsch. Med. Wschr. *107*: 1227−1231 (1982).

(19) WEIDNER, W., H. EBNER: Zytologische Analyse des Exprimaturins − Eine neue Möglichkeit zur Klassifikation der Prostatitis? In: BRUNNER, H., W. KRAUSE, C. F. ROTHAUGE, W. WEIDNER (eds.): Chronische Prostatitis; S. 173−182. Schattauer, Stuttgart−New York 1983a.

(20) WEIDNER, W., M. ARENS, H. KRAUSS, H. G. SCHIEFER, H. EBNER: Chlamydia trachomatis in "abacterial" prostatitis: microbiological, cytological and serological studies. Urologia internationalis *38*: 146−149 (1983b).

*Institut für Hygiene und Infektionskrankheiten der Tiere, Arbeitsgruppe Zoonosen,
Institut für Medizinische Mikrobiologie, Urologische Klinik, Zentrum für Pathologie,
Zytologisches Labor, der Universität Gießen*

Significance of Chlamydia trachomatis in "Abacterial" Prostatitis*

H. Krauss, H. G. Schiefer, W. Weidner, M. Arens, H. Ebner

Abstract

Chlamydia (C.) trachomatis was isolated in McCoy cell cultures from urethral swabs after prostatic massage, of 43 out of 233 patients (18.5%) with
symptoms of "abacterial" prostatitis, but also from 5 out of 65 control persons
(7.7%). Numbers of granulocytes in sediments of cytocentrifuged urine voided
after prostatic massage were normal (≤ 2, magn. 400×) in all 65 control persons, but were increased in 26 out of 43 patients with symptoms of "abacterial"
prostatitis (≥ 4, magn. 400×). Using an (H + L) chain specific anti-IgG FITC
conjugate, microimmunofluorescence tests for detection of antibodies against
C. trachomatis could be performed with the sera of all 65 control persons and
with those of 37 out of the 43 patients. All control persons, even those five with
positive *C. trachomatis* culture, were serologically negative (titer $< 1:8$), while
in 13 out of 15 *C. trachomatis* positive patients with a definitive diagnosis of
"abacterial" prostatitis, humoral antibodies with titers of $\geq 1:8$, predominantly
against serotypes I, J, E, and G, were detected. Serological results correlated
well with granulocyte counts in urines after prostatic massage. Patients with
symptoms of "abacterial" prostatitis with normal granulocyte counts (≤ 2) and
negative serology (titer $< 1:8$) were considered suffering from "prostatodynia".

Introduction

Chlamydia (C.) trachomatis is regarded to be one of the most important
agents of sexually transmitted diseases. 40 to 50% of cases of non-gonococcal
urethritis (NGU) or post-gonococcal urethritis (PGU) may be attributed to an

---

* This paper is originally published in „*Zentralblatt für Bakteriologie und Hygiene*", I. Abt. Orig.
A, *254*: 545−551 (1983), and is printed by permission of G. Fischer Verlag, Stuttgart.

infection with serotypes D−K of *C. trachomatis* (12). In patients under 40 years old and not suffering from lower urinary tract obstruction, *C. trachomatis* is supposed to be the most common agent of "abacterial" epididymitis (4).

"Abacterial" or "non-bacterial" prostatitis, clearly the most common type of prostatitis seen today (7), is an inflammation of the prostate characterized by high numbers of granulocytes in prostatic secretion, without conventional bacteria (3, 7). The significance of *C. trachomatis* in "abacterial" prostatitis has not been elucidated yet. Recent investigations in men with prostatitis in Canada (2), and Sweden (9), resulted in similar isolation rates as in NGU.

Since several years we have isolated *C. trachomatis* from men with NGU or PGU, as well as from patients with "abacterial" prostatitis (17). In this paper we report on observations concerning the relationships between results of clinical investigations in men with "abacterial" prostatitis, isolation of *C. trachomatis,* and development of specific antibodies against *C. trachomatis.*

Patients, materials and methods

Patients: 233 men with non-acute prostatitis (18−67 years old) and 65 healthy control persons (18−60 years of age), with an insignificant difference in the mean age of the two groups, were examined. All patients attended "Prostatitis-Sprechstunde", Urologische Klinik, Justus-Liebig-Universität Gießen.

Clinical Examination: In all patients, anamnestic exploration, digital prostatic examination, and uroflowmetric screening, was performed as described elsewhere (15).

Microbiological Investigations: Investigations for bacteria, mycoplasmas, chlamydiae, fungi, and *Trichomonas vaginalis* were performed using a standardized diagnostic procedure (11, 14, 16, 17) according to the "four specimens technique" (8). Only patients with symptoms of prostatitis and a monoinfection by *C. trachomatis* were included in this study.

Isolation of Chlamydia trachomatis: C. trachomatis was isolated from urethral swabs after standardized prostatic massage, or prostatic fluid (EPS), in McCoy cells cultivated on coverslips (10, 17). After incubation for three days, cells were fixed with methanol and stained after GIMÉNEZ. Inclusions appeared red on a green background. For positive diagnosis, at least two inclusions per coverslip were required.

Serology: The microimmunofluorescence (MIF) test for chlamydial antibodies (13) was slightly modified and used for detection of antibodies in patients' sera. Microscopic slides were covered with a thin film of Cariflex, a rubberlike product of Shell, and 16 antigen dots including all known 15 serotypes of *C. trachomatis* (originally obtained from the WHO Reference Center,

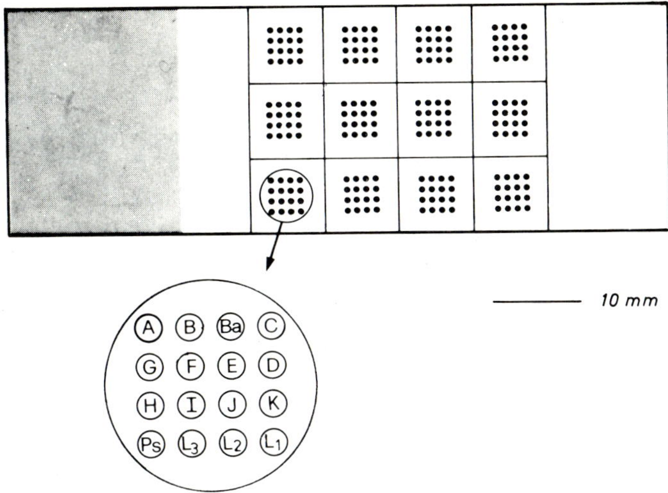

Fig. 1. Diagram of microimmunofluorescence test on slides; placement of 16 antigens per cluster.

London), plus a pool of four strains of *C. psittaci,* all propagated in McCoy cells, and finally adjusted to 10^7-10^8 organisms/ml, were placed in squares of 4×4 mm using a pen tip. By this technique two sera, each in six twofold dilutions from 1:8 to 1:256, could be studied using only one slide, thus minimizing antigen consumption (Fig. 1). A commercially available fluorescein-isothiocyanate-labeled rabbit IgG-conjugate against heavy and light chains of human IgG (Institut Pasteur), diluted 1:100 just before use, and combined with 5% Rhodamine counterstain (Difco), was applied. The dilution of serum, exhibiting a distinct particular fluorescence with at least one antigen of *C. trachomatis,* was called the titer. Titers of $\geq 1:8$ were regarded positive (1).

Cytological Analysis: Identical aliquots (3 ml) of midstream urine (VB2) and urine after prostatic massage (VB3) of all men were cytocentrifuged, the sedimented material transferred to a slide, and stained after Papanicolaou (18). When VB2 samples were free of leucocytes (≤ 2), the total number of polymorphonuclear leucocytes (PML) in VB3 was determined in 5 areas using a $400\times$ magnification. ≤ 2 PML/microscopic field were regarded as normal, ≤ 4 as borderline value, and > 4 PML as pathognomonic for prostatitis.

Statistics: Statistical analysis of differences in numbers was performed according to the test for analysis of differences in percentual numbers.

Results

C. trachomatis was isolated as sole agent from urethral swabs after prostatic massage in 43 (18.5%) of 233 patients with symptoms of prostatitis. However, *C. trachomatis* could also be isolated from 5 (7.7%) of 65 healthy control persons. Statistically the difference is significant on the 5%-level.

In none of the 65 control persons, i.e. also in none of the five healthy, but chlamydia-positive men, were elevated numbers of PML observed in cytocentrifuged urine after prostatic massage. In contrast, in 26 of 43 chlamydia-positive patients with prostatitis, >2 PML were found: in six men ≤4 PML, and in 20 men >4 PML per microscopic field were detected (Table 1).

Table 1. Polymorphonuclear granulocytes in sediments of cytocentrifuged urine after prostatic massage (VB3), in patients with mono-infection by *C. trachomatis* and symptoms of prostatitis, and in healthy control persons.

Patients (n = 43)	Control Persons (n = 65)	Polymorphonuclear Granulocytes in VB3 (Magn. × 400)	
11	48	None	Normal Range
6	17	≤ 2	
6	–	≤ 4	Borderline Range
13	–	≤10	Pathologic Range
3	–	≤20	
4	–	>20	

Sera of 37 of 43 men with chlamydia-positive prostatitis, and all sera of 65 control persons were studied in the MIF test. All sera were numbered, and while the investigator had no knowledge of the disease status of the test persons, results were compiled only after testing all sera available. Taking a titer of ≥1:8 as "positive", all control persons, including those with a positive culture of *C. trachomatis* from prostatic secretions, were serologically negative. Results of MIF tests with sera of the 37 patients with prostatitis and positive culture of *C. trachomatis* from prostatic secretions, correlated well with results of the cytological analysis of urines after prostatic massage, i.e., numbers of granulocytes. Humoral antibodies (IgG or IgM, since the conjugate was directed against heavy and light chains) with titers ≥1:8 against at least one type of *C. trachomatis,* mostly against several or even many types, and predominantly against types I, J, E, and G, were detected in the sera of 13 of 15 chlamydia-positive patients with highly elevated numbers of PML in urine after prostatic massage. Only two of these 15 men were serologically negative. In all patients with positive culture of *C. trachomatis* and insignificant numbers of PML (≤ 2 per microscopic field), no antibodies against *C. trachomatis* (titer $< 1:8$) were detected. Two out of 6 chlamydia-positive prostatitis patients with borderline values of PML had titers of 1:8, 4 of 6 were serologically negative (Table 2).

Table 2. Presence of humoral antibodies against *C. trachomatis* (MIF test), and granulocytes in sediments of cytocentrifuged urine after prostatic massage (VB3), in 37 patients with mono-infection by *C. trachomatis* and symptoms of prostatitis.

Patients (n = 37)	MIF-Negative ($< 1:8$)	MIF-Positive ($\geq 1:8$)	Polymorphonuclear Granulocytes in VB3 (Magnification $\times 400$)	
11	11	–	None	Normal Range
5	5	–	≤ 2	
6	4	2	≤ 4	Borderline Range
10	2	8	≤ 10	Pathologic Range
3	–	3	≤ 20	
2	–	2	> 20	

Table 3. Results of a follow-up study of a patient with mono-infection by *C. trachomatis* and urogenital disease: after diagnosis of NGU, development of prostatitis under tetracycline therapy, ending up with prostatodynia.

Disease	Date	Tetra-cycline Therapy	Isolation of *C. trachomatis*	Granulocytes in VB3 (Magnification $\times 400$)	MIF Test Titer/ Antigen
NGU	10/80	+	+ (Urethral Discharge)	> 10 (1. Voided Urine)	1:32/H
"Abacterial" Prostatitis	11/80	+	+ (EPS)	> 20 (VB3)	1:16/I
	3/81	+	+ (EPS)	≤ 10 (VB3)	1:16/J
	3/81	+	+ (EPS)	≤ 4 (VB3)	1:8/J
	3/81	+	– (EPS)	≤ 2 (VB3)	1:8/J, H
Prostatodynia	4/81	–	– (EPS)	– (VB3)	–/–

EPS = prostatic secretion; VB3 = cytocentrifuged urine after prostatic massage.

There were statistically highly significant correlations ($\alpha = 0.01$) between positive MIF tests and high numbers of PML in urine after prostatic massage, and negative serology and normal PML values, respectively.

In four chlamydia-positive patients with "abacterial" prostatitis following NGU, follow-up studies could be performed during and after treatment with tetracycline. Here also a remarkable correlation was found between presence of *C. trachomatis* in urethral discharge or urethral swabs after p. m., numbers of PML in urine after prostatic massage, and detection of specific antibodies against *C. trachomatis* with titers $\geq 1:8$ in the immunofluorescence test. In Table 3, these facts are demonstrated by the results of a follow-up study of one patient. Under prolonged treatment, isolation findings of *C. trachomatis* eventually became negative, leucocytes in urine after p. m. vanished, and antibodies subsided below a detectable level. However, the patient still complained of typical symptoms of prostatitis; then the disease was diagnosed as "prostatodynia" (symptoms of prostatitis without infection).

Discussion

In 1972, MÅRDH et al. (5) detected a serum complement fixing antibody titer of $\geq 1:5$ against chlamydia in 33% of 79 men with non-acute prostatitis, compared to 3% of 72 blood donors matched for age. In another investigation, using MIF test and cultural methods, MÅRDH et al. (6) obtained contradicting results, and suggested that *C. trachomatis* plays a minor, if any, etiological role in non-acute prostatitis. However, the patients they studied at that time had generally suffered from their disease for several years, and had received therapy with tetracyclines. *C. trachomatis* was isolated only in one of 53 patients.

BRUCE et al. (2) cultured early morning urine samples and/or prostatic fluid or semen and isolated *C. trachomatis* in 39 of 70 men (56%) with chronic prostatitis, compared to one of 50 normal men (2%). In the study by NILSSON et al. (9), 26 out of 96 men with symptoms of acute urethritis were harbouring *C. trachomatis* in the urethra but also had positive chlamydial cultures and a raised leucocyte count in their prostatic secretions. These findings indicated that *C. trachomatis* may be involved in the early inflammatory process engaging the prostate as a complication to nongonococcal urethritis.

In our investigation, detection of *C. trachomatis* in prostatic secretions or urethral swabs after prostatic massage of men with so-called "abacterial" prostatitis correlated well with the presence of specific humoral antibodies, even in follow-up studies of such patients. In cases of prostatodynia, which is characterized by negative bacteriology and low numbers of polymorphonuclear granulocytes in prostatic secretions (3, 7), isolation of *C. trachomatis* was rarely accompanied by development of specific chlamydial antibodies. While in "abacterial" prostatitis mere isolation of *C. trachomatis* from urethral swabs after prostatic massage or prostatic secretions does not provide conclusive evidence that chlamydia are involved in the disease, our findings indicate that *C. trachomatis* may indeed be incriminated as a causative agent of prostatitis, presumably as a consequence of chlamydial nongonococcal urethritis.

Acknowledgement

The support of Fraunhofer-Gesellschaft, München, ist gratefully acknowledged.

References

(1) ARENS, M., H. KRAUSS, H. G. SCHIEFER, W. WEIDNER, M. POPOVIC, M. SOBHY: Serologische Untersuchungen bei Patienten mit *C. trachomatis*-Infektionen des Urogenitaltraktes. In: ROTHAUGE, C. F., W. KRAUSE, W. WEIDNER (eds.): Chronische Prostatitis; p. 14. Schnetztor, Konstanz 1981.

(2) BRUCE, A. W., P. CHADWICK, W. S. WILLETT, M. O'SHAUGNESSY: The role of chlamydia in genito-urinary disease. J. Urol. *126*: 625−629 (1981).

(3) DRACH, G. W., E. M. MEARES, W. R. FAIR, T. A. STAMEY: Classification of benign diseases associated with prostatic pain: prostatitis or prostatodynia? J. Urol. *120*: 266 (1978).

(4) HARNISCH, J. P., R. E. BERGER, E. R. ALEXANDER, G. MONDA, K. K. HOLMES: Etiology of acute epididymitis. Lancet *I*: 819−821 (1977).

(5) MÅRDH, P.-A., S. COLLEEN, B. HOLMQUIST: Chlamydia in chronic prostatitis. Brit. Med. J. *IV*: 361 (1972).

(6) MÅRDH, P.-A., K. T. RIPA, S. COLLEEN, J. D. TREHARNE, S. DAROUGAR: Role of *Chlamydia trachomatis* in non-acute prostatitis. Brit. J. vener. Dis. *54*: 330−334 (1978).

(7) MEARES, E. M.: Prostatitis syndromes: perspectives about old woes. J. Urol. *123*: 141−147 (1980).

(8) MEARES, E. M., T. A. STAMEY: Bacteriologic localization patterns in bacterial prostatitis and urethritis. Invest. Urol. *5*: 492−518 (1968).

(9) NILSSON, S., G. JOHANNISSON, E. LYCKE: Isolation of *Chlamydia trachomatis* from the urethra and from prostatic fluid in men with signs and symptoms of acute urethritis. Acta derm.-venereol. *61*: 456−459 (1981).

(10) RIPA, K. T., P.-A. MÅRDH: Cultivation of *C. trachomatis* in cycloheximide-treated McCoy cells. J. clin. Microbiol. *6*: 328−331 (1977).

(11) SCHIEFER, H. G., W. WEIDNER, H. KRAUSS, U. GERHARDT, K. L. SCHMIDT: Rheumatoid Factor-Negative Arthritis, especially Ankylosing Spondylitis, and Infections of the Male Urogenital Tract. Zbl. Bakt. Hyg., I. Abt. Orig. A *255*: 511−517 (1983).

(12) TAYLOR-ROBINSON, D., B. J. THOMAS: The rôle of Chlamydia trachomatis in genital-tract and associated diseases. J. clin. Path. *33*: 205−233 (1980).

(13) WANG, W. P., J. T. GRAYSTON, E. R. ALEXANDER, K. K. HOLMES: Simplified microimmunofluorescence test with Trachoma-Lymphogranuloma venereum *(Chlamydia trachomatis)* antigens for use as screening test for antibody. J. clin. Microbiol. *1*: 250−255 (1975).

(14) WEIDNER, W., H. BRUNNER, W. KRAUSE, C. F. ROTHAUGE: Zur Bedeutung von *Ureaplasma urealyticum* bei unspezifischer Prostato-Urethritis. Dtsch. med. Wschr. *103*: 465−470 (1978).

(15) WEIDNER, W., H. BRUNNER, W. KRAUSE, R. PUST: *Ureaplasma urealyticum* bei chronischer unspezifischer Prostato-Urethritis. Akt. Urol. *10*: 1−7 (1979).

(16) WEIDNER, W., H. BRUNNER, W. KRAUSE: Quantitative culture of *Ureaplasma urealyticum* in patients with chronic prostatitis or prostatosis. J. Urol. *124*: 622−625 (1980).

(17) WEIDNER, W., H. G. SCHIEFER, H. KRAUSS, J. ENGSTFELD: Untersuchungen zur Ätiologie der nicht-gonorrhoischen Urethritis. Dtsch. med. Wsch. *107*: 1227−1231 (1982).

(18) WEIDNER, W., H. EBNER: Zytologische Analyse des Exprimaturins auf Entzündungszellen − eine neue Möglichkeit zur Klassifizierung der Prostatitis. In: ROTHAUGE, C. F., W. KRAUSE, W. WEIDNER (eds.): Chronische Prostatitis; p. 25. Schnetztor, Konstanz 1981.

*Andrology Unit, Urology Department, Microbiology Department, Pathology Department
of the Hospital of Magenta, Milano*

Bacterial Flora in Expressed Prostatic and Vesicular Secretions of Infertile Subjects

G. M. COLPI, A. ZANOLLO, M. ROVEDA, A. TOMMASINI-DEGNA, G. BERETTA

Abstract

A bacteriological study was performed on prostatic (EPS) and vesicular (EVS) secretions from 123 infertile men who were suspected of having chronic genital tract inflammation and from 31 men with premature ejaculation. Samples were inoculated within 10 min on various culture media and incubated under both aerobic and anaerobic conditions. Bacterial numbers of more than 10,000 colony-forming units of a single species or genus per ml of EPS or EVS were considered to be pathological.

In the infertile subjects with proven inflammation of the seminal accessory glands, the EPS and the EVS that gave positive cultures and had bacterial numbers defined as pathological contained large numbers of anaerobic or microaerophilic organisms (EPS: 51 of the 63 bacterial strains found, $\simeq 81\%$; EVS: 19 of the 20 bacterial strains found, $\simeq 95\%$).

Introduction

Many investigators have studied the microbial flora of the seminal tract in men of fertile age by culturing ejaculate samples. It has been stated that semen samples from virgin subjects usually contain no bacteria (7) and those from fertile men contain only a few (8, 16, 17, 20), while those of most infertile men, even when they have no symptoms of infection, often have variable amounts of more than one bacterial strain at the same time (4, 11, 15, 17, 19).

In an attempt to determine whether these bacteria come from the prostate or the seminal vesicles, the ejaculate has been split roughly into prostatic and vesicular fractions and these have been cultured separately (12).

However, germs present on the urethral walls might well be sloughed off during ejaculation (9) and distributed non uniformly throughout the seminal fluid: therefore the method used is not free of error. In addition, collection of ejaculate by masturbation, even under the most sterile conditions possible, is not completely free of risk of contamination and might thus give misleading results.

In order to gain more information about the specific microbial flora of the prostate and of the seminal vesicles in infertile men, we have studied the aerobic and anaerobic bacteria in samples of secretion obtained by direct massage of those glands.

Materials and methods

Our patient population consisted of 123 infertile men aged from 23 to 50 years (mean age: 33.2 ± 5.3 years) whose medical histories (frequency of urination, dysuria, prostatorrhea) and/or physical findings (prostatic congestion, or induration and irregularity, or tenderness) and/or seminological data (abnormal liquefaction, constant hyperviscosity, leukospermia ($>10^6$ WBC/ml), pseudoagglutination and/or asthenozoospermia) caused us to suspect the existence of chronic seminal tract inflammation. Forty-four men were asthenozoospermic, 13 oligoasthenozoospermic, 22 asthenoteratozoospermic, 33 oligoasthenoteratozoospermic, 8 azoospermic and 3 aspermic.

Our controls were 31 subjects who either had normal sperm samples or were fathers, aged from 20 to 46 years (mean age: 27.7 ± 6.5 years), who complained of premature ejaculation.

We first examined the ejaculate of each subject after sexual abstinence for 3−5 days. Then 7 to 15 days later, including an additional period of sexual abstinence of 7 days and abstention from urination for 4−8 hours, samples were obtained by prostatic and, when possible, vesicular massage, using a modified Meares and Stamey method (18) (Fig. 1).

The glans was very carefully cleaned with sterile gauze and Bialcool™ (Ciba-Geigy, Basel, Switzerland) and the prepuce was held back throughout sample collection. The patient was asked to partly empty his bladder and to collect a sample of 5−10 ml of urine from the mid-stream fraction (VB2). The patient was then placed in the genu-cubital position. In this position the examiner can best palpate the seminal vesicles with the forefinger of one hand and use the other hand to press over the partly full bladder; and the flow along the urethra of the expressed prostatic and the expressed vesicular secretions is facilitated. They are collected by gravity, minimizing the risks of external contamination.

The glans was again disinfected and the subject's prostate was massaged. The first one or two drops of prostatic secretion were discarded and one drop was then collected for the microbiological investigation, one drop for the cy-

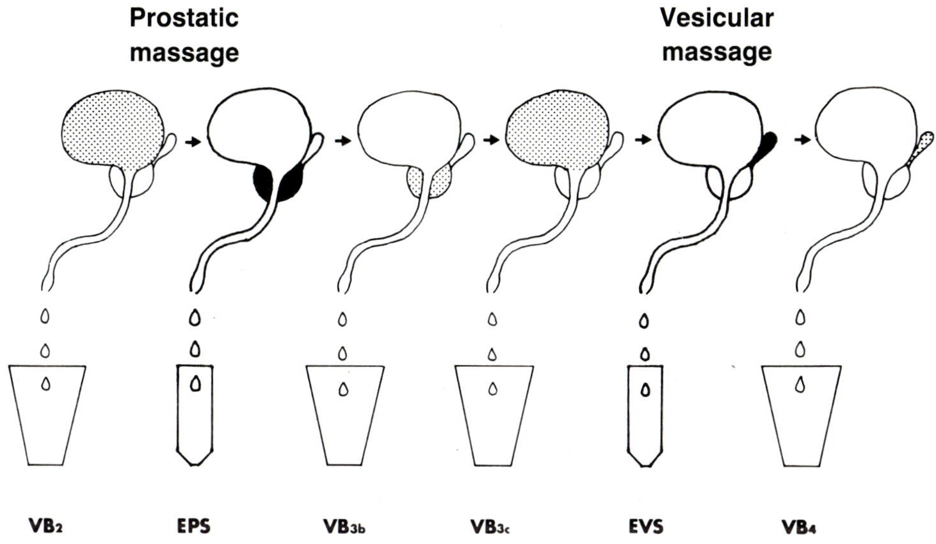

VB2   : "voided bladder" (pre-massage).
EPS   : expressed prostatic secretion (by prostatic massage).
VB3b   : early voided bladder (after prostatic massage).
VB3c   : late voided bladder.
EVS   : expressed vesicular secretion (by vesicular massage).
VB4   : early voided bladder (after vesicular massage).

Fig. 1. Samples collected. [Modified from MEARES and STAMEY (16).]

tological investigation and another drop for the biochemical tests (EPS) (18). After the prostatic massage, the patient was again asked to partially empty his bladder and to collect the first 2−5 ml (VB3b) and the last 5−10 ml of urine (VB3c) for microbiological and cytological tests.

After a third disinfection of the glans, the subject's seminal vesicles were massaged. The first drop was discarded and any drops of vesicular secretion (EVS) that could be obtained were collected for microbiological, cytological and biochemical investigations. The first 2−3 ml of urine voided after vesicular massage (VB4) were always collected for microbiological and cytological investigations. In clinical practice this usually enables us to examine vesicular secretion (diluted in urine), which in itself is viscous and does not always emerge from the urethral meatus during vesicular massage. It is not easy to obtain samples of EVS. One needs an experienced investigator, a thin patient, not too stocky, with a pelvis that can easily be palpated rectally, but even this does not guarantee collection of pure EVS samples. In this study we will present only our data concerning pure samples of EVS.

For microbiological investigation samples were inoculated within 10 minutes of collection into the following culture media: Blood agar, Endo agar (selective for Enterobacteria), Mannitol salt agar (selective for Staphylococci), Schaedler Agar + vitamin K + 5% sheep blood, Kanamycin-Vancomycin Agar + 5% sheep blood, PPLO agar + growth factors (selective for Mycoplasmas and L-forms), with distribution of 10 or 20 µl of material with a calibrated bacteriological loop, going from the first to the fourth quadrant of each plate. The plates were incubated aerobically and anaerobically (in a Gas Pak Jar System, BBL) at 37°C for 48 hrs; these of PPLO agar were incubated in 5% CO_2 for 4 days. The aerobic microorganisms were identified and a Kirby-Bauer antibiogram was made. The anaerobic organisms were described morphologically and their Gram-stain characteristics determined. The colonies growing on the culture media were counted and the numbers of colony-forming units per ml in the original specimens were then calculated.

Other samples of EPS were examined cytologically by the method of ANDERSON and WELLER (1). Prostatic inflammation was considered to be of clinical significance when there were more than 1,000 inflammatory elements/mm³ of EPS.

Biochemical investigation consisted of high-resolution electrophoresis of the proteins in the EPS and EVS samples (3).

Results and discussion

We do not know the minimal bacterial numbers to be considered pathological, i. e. indicating infection. It is usually considered that the numbers in EPS are pathological if they are greater than in VB2 (18). There are no data at all in the literature for the EVS. For ejaculate collected under the most sterile conditions possible, a contemporary growth of two or more species of bacteria in different numbers is not at all rare (4, 11, 15, 19) and bacterial numbers of more than 10,000 colony-forming units/ml for Gram-positive and of less than that for Gram-negative bacteria are considered pathological (2, 20). We chose cut-off points for EPS and EVS of more than 10,000 colonies/ml as pathological (M+), and more than 3,000 colonies/ml of a single bacterial species or genus as suspicious (M±) when the cytology was also pathological. If the urine (VB2 and VB3b) contained more than 3,000 colonies/ml, the EPS and EVS numbers were not considered to indicate prostatic or vesicular infection.

Table 1 lists the results of the microbiological investigations of the EPS and the cytology, for the infertile subjects and the controls. The different incidence of the pathological microbiological findings, analyzed statistically by the Chi-square test, was significant (p < 0.01).

Table 1. Distribution of the infertile subjects and of the controls according to the combined results of the microbiological and cytological investigations of the EPS.

	Infertile subjects		Controls	
M+ C+	15	(12.2%)	0	(0.0%)
M+ C−	21	(17.1%)	1	(3.2%)
M± C+	7	(5.7%)	1	(3.2%)
M− C+	25	(20.3%)	4	(12.9%)
M− C−	55	(44.7%)	25	(80.7%)
Total	123	(100.0%)	31	(100.0%)

M+ and M−: respectively indicate microbiological findings positive and negative for a prostatic infection.

M±: indicates microbiological suspicious finding in presence of a cytological positive finding.

C+ and C−: respectively indicate cytological findings positive and negative for a prostatic inflammation.

Table 2. Bacteria isolated from the EPS of 43 infertile subjects with significant bacterial numbers.

	M+	M±	Total
Staphylococci	2	1	3
Streptococci	3	1	4
Micrococci	2	–	2
E. coli	3	–	3
Proteus	1	–	1
Mycoplasmas and L-forms	1	–	1
Microaerophilic Gram + bacilli	10	2	12
Anaerobic Gram + bacilli	6	1	7
Anaerobic Gram + cocci	13	1	14
Anaerobic Gram − bacilli	12	–	12
Anaerobic Gram − cocci	10	1	11

EPS with pathological bacterial numbers (M+): 36
EPS with "suspicious bacterial numbers (M±):   7
Strains isolated: 70
  − aerobes   14 (20.0%)
  − microaerophils   12 (17.0%)
  − anaerobes   44 (63.0%)

Note: The first two columns respectively indicate the numbers of cases in which the same bacterial species or genus was isolated independently from the cytological findings in numbers of more than 10,000 colony-forming units/ml (M+), and in numbers of more than 3,000 colony-forming units/ml in presence of a positive cytological finding (M±).

Table 2 lists the bacteria isolated from 43 infertile men whose EPS cultures were considered pathological or suspicious. Of the 70 bacterial strains isolated, 14 were aerobes ($\simeq 20.0\%$), 12 were microaerophiles ($\simeq 17.0\%$) and 44 were anaerobes ($\simeq 63.0\%$).

The seminal vesicles of all 123 infertile subjects were massaged, but only 27 pure EVS samples could be obtained. Unlike EPS, which is quite liquid, EVS is opalescent, sometimes gelatinous and always rather viscous. It consists of vesicular secretion, possibly contaminated by secretion of ampullar origin. So, under the microscope, one can see spermatozoa, cells of variable morphology from the seminal vesicles epithelium (13), cell detritus and sometimes immature germ cells and leukocytes (5). After preliminary evaluation on this basis, the purity of the apparently pure EVS samples was further checked by high-resolution electrophoresis of the proteins. The protein patterns of EPS and EVS are characteristic and very different (3), and this method eliminated impure samples of EVS.

Table 3 shows the microbiological findings for the EVS and the EPS samples from the 27 infertile subjects. Fourteen of 27 subjects had pathological bacterial numbers. Of these, 8 also had pathological EPS numbers with the same counts and species in 6, different in 2; six had negative microbiology. Only 1 of the 13 subjects with negative EVS had a positive EPS. This is contrary to the current opinion, that the prostate is the defense organ against ascending infection of the seminal tract, which would require the prostate to be infected when the seminal vesicles are. However, this may be an artefact due to the greater ease of vesicular massage, when there is vesiculitis.

Finally Table 4 lists the bacteria isolated from the EVS samples of the 14 infertile subjects with pathological bacterial numbers. Of the 20 bacterial strains, 1 was an L-form ($\simeq 5\%$), 3 were microaerophiles ($\simeq 15\%$) and 16 were anaerobes ($\simeq 80\%$).

Table 3. Microbiological findings for the EVS and EPS samples from the 27 infertile men from whom pure samples of EVS were obtained.

EVS		EPS	No.
M+	=	M+	6
M+	≠	M+	2
M+		M−	6
M−		M+	1
M−		M−	12
Total			27

Table 4. Bacteria isolated from the EVS of 14 infertile subjects with pathological bacterial numbers.

	No.
Staphylococci	–
Streptococci	–
Micrococci	–
E. coli	–
Proteus	–
L-forms	1
Microaerophilic Gram + bacilli	3
Anaerobic Gram + bacilli	1
Anaerobic Gram + cocci	4
Anaerobic Gram – bacilli	6
Anaerobic Gram – cocci	5

Strains isolated: 20
- aerobes　　　　1 (5.0%)
- microaerophils　3 (15.0%)
- anaerobes　　　16 (80.0%)

Conclusion

We found increased numbers of anaerobic or microaerophilic bacteria in male accessory genital gland secretions of infertile subjects (51 bacterial strains of 63 isolated from EPS, $\simeq 81\%$; 19 bacterial strains of 20 isolated from EVS, $\simeq 95\%$). This indicates to us that search for anaerobic bacteria should be added to routine clinical examination of whole ejaculate, split ejaculate or EPS samples, when seminal tract infection is suspected.

References

(1) ANDERSON, R. U., C. WELLER: Prostatic secretion leukocyte studies in non-bacterial prostatitis (prostatosis). J. Urol. *121*: 292–294 (1979).

(2) ARVIS, G.: Sperme et prostatite chronique. In: HENRY-SUCHET, J., A. STEG, A. CONSTANTIN (eds.): Infection et Fécondité; pp. 27–32. Masson, Paris 1977.

(3) BALERNA, M., G. M. COLPI, A. CAMPANA, M. L. ROVEDA, A. TOMMASINI-DEGNA, A. ZANOLLO: High-resolution protein patterns of human expressed prostatic secretion: a new tool for the diagnosis of prostatitis. Arch. Androl. *8*: 97–105 (1982).

(4) BRUN, B., J. P. BISSON, A. CLAVERT: Modifications des caractéristiques du sperme en présence de germs. In: HENRY-SUCHET, J., A. STEG, A. CONSTANTIN (eds.): Infection et Fécondité; pp. 33–42. Masson, Paris 1977.

(5) COLPI, G. M., A. LANGÉ: Le "Round Cells" nel Liquido Seminale; pp. 23–90. Cofese, Palermo 1977.

(6) COMHAIRE, F., G. VERSCHRAEGEN, L. VERMEULEN: Diagnosis of accessory gland infection and its possible role in male infertility. Int. J. Androl. *3*: 32−45 (1980).

(7) DAHLBERG, B.: Asymptomatic bacteriospermia. Urologia *8*: 563 (1976).

(8) DERRICK, F. C., JR., B. DAHLBERG: Male genital tract infections and sperm viability. In: HAFEZ, E. S. E. (ed.): Human Semen and Fertility Regulation in Men; pp. 389−397. Mosby, St. Louis 1976.

(9) DESAI, S., M. S. COHEN, M. KHATAMEE, E. LEITER: Ureaplasma urealyticum (T-mycoplasma) infection: does it have a role in male infertility? J. Urol. *124*: 469−471 (1980).

(10) ELIASSON, R.: Clinical examination of infertile men. In: HAFEZ, E. S. E. (ed.): Human Semen and Fertility Regulation in Men; pp. 321−331. Mosby, St. Louis 1976.

(11) ENEROTH, P., Å. LJUNGH-WADSTRÖM, P. J. MOBERG, C.-E. NORD: Studies on the bacterial flora in semen from males in infertile relations. Int. J. Androl. *1*: 105−116 (1978).

(12) FARI, A., R. TRÉVOUX, J. VERGÉS, J. BELAISCH, J. LAFARGE: Incidence des états inflammatoires ou infectieux des glandes génitales annexes sur le sperme. In: HENRY-SUCHET, J., A. STEG, A. CONSTANTIN (eds.): Infection et Fécondité; pp. 43−58. Masson, Paris 1977.

(13) LANGÉ, A., G. M. COLPI, M. GIUDICI, A. TOMMASINI-DEGNA: Le cellule provenienti dalle vescicole seminali negli strisci da puntato prostatico transrettale, da massaggio prostatico e di liquido seminale: diagnostica differenziale e correlazione cito-istologica. Atti LI° Congr. Soc. Ital. Urologia *II*: 97−112 (1978).

(14) MEARES, E. M., JR.: Prostatitis syndromes: new perspectives about old woes. J. Urol. *123*: 141−147 (1980).

(15) MOBERG, P. J., P. ENEROTH, Å. LJUNG, C.-E. NORD: Bacterial flora in semen before and after doxycycline treatment of infertile couples. Int. J. Androl. *3*: 46−58 (1980).

(16) MOBLEY, D. F.: Semen cultures in the diagnosis of bacterial prostatitis. J. Urol. *114*: 83−85 (1975).

(17) REHEWY, M. S., E. S. E. HAFEZ, A. THOMAS, W. J. BROWN: Aerobic and anaerobic bacterial flora in semen from fertile and infertile groups of men. Arch. Androl. *2*: 263−268 (1979).

(18) STAMEY, T. A.: Urinary Infections. Chaps. 1; 7. Williams & Wilkins, Baltimore 1972.

(19) SWENSON, CH. E., A. TOTH, CL. TOTH, L. WOLFGRUBER, W. M. O'LEARY: Asymptomatic bacteriospermia in infertile men. Andrologia *12*: 7−11 (1980).

(20) ULSTEIN, M., P. CAPELL, K. K. HOLMES, C. A. PAULSEN: Nonsymptomatic genital tract infection and male infertility. In: HAFEZ, E. S. E. (ed.): Human Semen and Fertility Regulation in Men; pp. 355−362. Mosby, St. Louis 1976.

Institut für Virologie der Universität Köln

Can Herpesvirus hominis be Isolated from the Genitourinary Tract of Men Having no Manifest Symptoms of Herpesvirus Infection?*

TH. MERTENS, A. LANVERS, H. J. EGGERS

Quite a number of viruses are capable of producing a wide spectrum of disease manifestations in human beings. Herpes simplex virus (HSV) is one of them. HSV may cause, for example, fatal encephalitis, recurring facial or genital herpes lesions, or even a primary infection without clinical signs at all. In the past, a variety of diseases, especially of the genitourinary tract, have been connected with herpes viruses.

Recurrent oral or genital infections which − as is well known − may be excruciating for the patients, do point to a special pathogenetic mechanism. There are mainly three hypotheses designed to explain recurring infections (EPSTEIN, 1976).

1. Exogenous or endogenous reinfection leads to consecutive herpes manifestations.
2. Primary herpes infection leads to chronic infection with a continuous, low grade virus production. Herpes simplex virus may exacerbate and produce recurrent clinical manifestations.
3. Primary infection produces latent infection of the corresponding neuron in sensory ganglia without any production of viral particles during the symptom-free interval.

Several cases have been reported in support of the first hypothesis. If a massive infection with HSV occurs, even seropositive persons can suffer an exogenous reinfection (e.g. nurses) (EPSTEIN, 1976). Especially in children endogenous reinfection has been reported, namely an autoinoculation from a primary efflorescence to another skin area (for example to the genitalia) (NAHMIAS et al., 1968). At this secondary inoculation site even recurrent herpes is possible.

* We very much appreciate the cooperation of Professor Dr. med. R. ENGELKING, Direktor der Urologischen Klinik der Universität Köln, Dr. med. H. D. LEHMANN, Chefarzt der Urologischen Abteilung des Städtischen Krankenhauses Holweide (Köln), and Professor Dr. med. G. K. STEIGLEDER, Direktor der Hautklinik der Universität Köln, for providing us with clinical specimens.

Nevertheless, reinfections do not appear to be the usual mechanism of recurrent herpes.

There is also very good evidence for the third hypothesis. In trigeminal and sacral ganglia of humans and animals herpes virus genomes have been detected in the absence of infectious virus, thus demonstrating latent infection (STEVENS, 1978; BARINGER and SWOVELAND, 1973; BARINGER, 1974). The mechanism of reactivation of the viral genome which might clinically lead to recurrence, is still unknown.

Let us now consider the second hypothesis which claims local persistence of HSV in *peripheral,* non-neural tissues, additionally to the well-established neural persistence. There is the following evidence supporting this hypothesis. First, data from animal experiments show local persistence at the peripheral inoculation site (*footpad* of guinea pigs) (SCRIBA, 1981). The other evidence consists of a number of reports, mainly from a single laboratory, of herpesvirus isolations (up to 20%) from the urogenital tract of asymptomatic males (DEARDOURFF et al., 1974).

If it is true, as hypothesis No. 2 claims that herpes virus is resident in and can be isolated from peripheral tissues of the genitourinary tract, even in asymptomatic man, it would be very difficult to clarify its etiological involvement in a number of genital diseases, including chronic prostatitis.

Considering the work of DEARDOURFF and his group, we were impressed by their high isolation rate which did not agree with the experience we had made in our routine diagnostic laboratory. Therefore, we tried to reproduce these results.

We attempted to isolate HSV from the genitourinary tract of 181 patients with urological or andrological symptoms but asymptomatic with regard to herpetic disease at the time of examination. Table 1 shows data of the patients investigated. It is grouped according to age of the patients and the clinical diagnosis which brought them to the hospital. The sixth column shows the percentages of HSV seropositive reactions in the different age groups which is in agreement with the literature. The last two columns contain the calculated numbers and percentages of positive isolations that would have to be expected according to DEARDOURFF et al. Special attention should be paid to the three patients with a history of genital herpes which figure under the marked diagnoses (see Table 1).

Table 2 presents our scurtinous virological procedures. The urethral swabs and seminal fluids were inoculated for virus isolation attempts into cultures of two cell lines both shown to be highly sensitive to herpes virus infection. Genitourinary tissue probes obtained freshly from urological operations were cut into halves: one piece was homogenized and inoculated into cultures of the two respective cell lines, the second piece was trypsinized and a suspension of

Table 1. Data of investigated patients.

Age group (years)	No.	Clinical diagnosis	History of Clinical herpes H.lab.	History of Clinical herpes H.genit.	Serum Pos. CF	Expected virus isolations** No.	Expected virus isolations** %
15–45	97	Infertility/ sterilisation 56* Prostatopathia/prostatitis/ epididymitis 6 Varicocele 6 others (urethritis)*	10	2*	69%	12.8	13.2
46–60	27	Prostatic adenoma 10 Tumour of the urinary bladder 4 Prostatitis/epididymitis 2* others	5	1*	96%	3.9	14.2
61–70	29	Prostatic adenoma 18 Prostatic carcinoma 6 others	1	0	79%	5.2	17.9
>70	28	Prostatic adenoma 17 Prostatic carcinoma 5 Tumour of the urinary bladder 3 others	1	0	75%	4.3	15.2
Total	181		17	3	75%	26.2	14.5

 * Herpes genitalis anamnesis.
** According to DEARDOURFF et al., 1974.

vital cells was cocultivated with an equal number of rabbit kidney cells. Eighteen of the cocultivated cell cultures were treated with polyethylene glycol (PEG) in order to induce cell fusion.

We should like to stress the fact that our material was processed within 3 hours under optimum conditions. We thus used the most sensitive procedures of demonstrating infectious virus at present available.

Table 3 summarizes our results. In the first column the specimens investigated are listed, in the next one the methods applied, then our own isolation results, and finally − for comparison − those that would have been expected according to DEARDOURFF et al.

Not in a single case we were able to isolate herpes virus. Thus, we have to answer the leading question of our study, viz. can evidence be found of herpes virus persistence in extraneural (peripheral) tissues of the genitourinary tract in asymptomatic males? There is *no* such evidence!

Table 2. Virological investigations.

Material	Methods
1. Urethral swabs	Cell culture: RK_{13}*, HEL**
2. Seminal fluids or prostatic exprimates	Cell culture: RK_{13}, HEL

3. Genitourinary tract tissue probes***
    a) 1st piece
 	
    b) 2nd piece
	Tissue homogenisation
	cell culture (RK_{13}, HEL)
	Co-cultivation (RK_{13})
	Cell fusion (RK_{13})

4. Blood serum	Complement fixation test

  * RK_{13} = permanent cell line derived from rabbit kidney.
 ** HEL = human embryonic lung fibroblasts. Both cell lines have been shown to be highly sensitive to herpesvirus infection.
*** Fresh material from urological operations was cut in halves.

Table 3. Results of isolation attemps.

Specimens investigated	No.	Methods of virus isolation			Positive virus isolations	Expected virus isolations*	
		Cell culture	Co-culti-vation	Fusion (PEG)		No.	%
Urethral swabs	89	89	–	–	0	6.8	7.6
Prostatic and seminal fluids	55	55	–	–	0	16.2	29.4
Tissues (total)	48	48	45	18	0	–	–
Prostatic adenoma	23	23	23	10	0	5.2	19.4
Prostatic carcinoma	4	4	4	2	0	–	–
Vas deferens	13	13	13	6	0	3.4	26.0
Other tissue probes, e. g.: Testes Bladder tumour Foreskin Ureter	8	8	5	–	0	1.2	15.3

* According to DEARDOURFF et al., 1974.

The fact that the male urogenital tract can not be considered normally as a reservoir of herpes virus, in our view, is crucial for the etiological interpretation of possible future herpes virus isolations in certain disease entities. Furthermore: asymptomatic males apparently play no role as vector for the transmission of herpes genitalis.

References

(1) Baringer, J. R., P. Swoveland: Recovery of herpes simplex virus from human trigeminal ganglions. New Engl. J. Med. *288*: 648−650 (1973).

(2) Baringer, J. R.: Recovery of herpes simplex virus from human sacral ganglions. New Engl. J. Med. *291*: 828−830 (1974).

(3) Deardourff, St. L., F. A. Deture, D. M. Drylie, Y. Centifano, H. Kaufman: Association between herpes hominis type 2 and the male genitourinary tract. J. Urol. *112*: 126−127 (1974).

(4) Epstein, W. S.: Latency in herpesvirus hominis: its relationship to oncogenesis and recurrent disease. Texas Medicine *72*: 84−94 (1976).

(5) Nahmias, A. J., W. R. Dowdle, Z. M. Naib, W. E. Josey, C. F. Luce: Genital infection with herpesvirus hominis types 1 and 2 in children. Pediatrics *42*: 659−666 (1968).

(6) Scriba, M.: Persistence of herpes simplex virus (HSV) infection in ganglia and peripheral tissues of guinea pigs. Med. Microbiol. Immunol. *169*: 91−96 (1981).

(7) Stevens, J. G.: Latent characteristics of selected herpesviruses. Adv. Cancer Res. *26*: 227−256 (1978).

Urology Section, Palo Alto Veterans Administration Medical Center, Palo Alto, Calif.
Division of Urology, Stanford University School of Medicine, Stanford, Calif.

The Immunologic Characterization of Bacterial Prostatitis Caused by Enterobacteriaceae

L. M. D. SHORTLIFFE, T. A. STAMEY

Introduction

Since it is known that bacterial and viral pathogens elicit a local secretory immune response at various human mucosal glandular surfaces, such as gastrointestinal, respiratory and vaginal mucosa, we decided to investigate whether a similar response could be detected from the prostate. We wished to establish whether we could measure local and systemic immune responses to prostatic infection and what the natural history to any existing responses would be. To do this, we studied the serum and prostatic fluid of patients with acute and chronic bacterial prostatitis, patients with nonbacterial prostatitis, and normal males who had no history of previous urinary tract infections. Specimens from two patients with bacterial prostatitis were collected at the time of infection and for two years afterwards.

Methods

Each patient had quantitative bacteriologic localization procedures to culture the urethra, voided urine, and prostatic secretions on each visit. Specimens were the first voided 5–10 ml urine (VB1), the midstream aliquot (VB2), the prostatic fluid produced from prostatic massage (EPS, expressed prostatic secretion), and the first 5–10 ml urine voided immediately after massage. These specimens were cultured for bacteria and frozen at $-70°$C. Simultaneous serum specimens were obtained from each patient. All significant organisms which were cultured were stored.

Both prostatic fluid and serum specimens were assayed for total and antigen-specific IgA and IgG. Total nonspecific immunoglobulins were measured by commercial radial immunodiffusion agar plates. Antigen-specific antibodies, those immunoglobulins formed against the infecting organisms, were measured using an indirect solid phase radioimmunoassay previously described by ZOL-LINGER and associates (1) which we modified to measure antibodies to Enterobacteriaceae (2). Formalin-fixed whole bacterial antigen was prepared from previously stored specimens at concentrations of 10^9 oragnisms/ml. Serial two-fold dilutions for each serum and EPS specimen were assayed in duplicate for IgA and IgG antigen-specific antibodies as follows. Formalin-fixed bacterial antigen was placed in the polyvinylchloride wells for 1 h at 37°C to cause adherence to this solid phase. The excess antigen was washed from the wells, and bovine serum albumin was placed into the wells as a filler to block further binding of materials to the solid phase. Excess albumin was washed out, and the specimen to be tested was placed into the well overnight at room temperature. This allowed the antigen-specific antibodies to bind to the bacterial antigen which was attached to the plastic solid phase. Excess unbound specimen was removed and an I^{125} labeled antihuman-immunoglobulin (either anti IgG or IgA) was placed into the well overnight. This antihuman immunoglobulin radioactively labeled the antigen-specific antibodies. Each well was placed in a test tube and radioactivity was measured by a gamma scintillation counter. When serial dilutions of specimens are assayed, a curve of the radioactivity measured at each dilution can be plotted. From this curve a dilution at which radioactivity will be proportional to the quantity of antigen-specific antibody present can be selected. The reciprocal of the specimen dilution which corresponds to a previously determined level of radioactivity was designated the antigen-specific antibody titer.

Similarly, total nonspecific immunoglobulin was measured in specimens by binding antihuman-immunoglobulin to the plastic solid phase. The specimen to be tested was placed in the well so that the antihuman immunoglobulin attached to the plastic could bind to immunoglobulin in the specimen. The excess specimen was removed and I^{125} labeled antihuman immunoglobulin was placed in the well again to label the previously bound immunoglobulin from the specimen. Both secretory and serum IgA could be detected using this assay.

Patients

Males without history of urinary tract infections, males with acute and chronic bacterial prostatitis, and males with nonbacterial prostatitis were studied. Two patients, one with acute bacterial prostatitis, and the other with chronic bacterial prostatitis were followed with longitudinal serum and prostatic specimens to study the natural history of their immune response to bacterial prostatic infection.

Patient 1 is a 45-year-old man who had a 6-year history of recurrent urinary tract infections and presented with symptoms of an acute prostatitis in 1973.

After treatment with ampicillin a lower tract bacterial localization study proved he had *E. coli 04* in his prostate. He was treated and cured with trimethoprim-sulfamethoxazole for 90 d. He was next seen in our urology clinic in December 1978, when he had 3 d of chills, dysuria, and elevated temperatures. After treatment with nitrofurantoin, a lower tract bacteriologic localization study showed *E. coli 018* in his prostate. His right prostatic lobe was rock-hard and multiple oval fat macrophages were seen in the prostatic fluid. He was treated with 90 d trimethoprim-sulfamethoxazole and all his symptoms disappeared. During this interval and the subsequent two years all cultures were sterile for any gram-negative organisms, and the prostatic examination reverted to normal.

Patient 2 is a 43-year-old man who had a laminectomy in 1971 and then wore an indwelling urethral catheter for three months. After removal of the catheter he developed recurrent urinary infections and epididymitis requiring a vasectomy to prevent further infections. He was first seen in our urology clinic in 1974 with *E. coli 01* bacteriuria. After treatment with trimethoprim-sulfamethoxazole he had persistent *E. coli 01* in his prostate until a prostatic calculus was found and removed. His cultures then remained sterile until 1976 when he was lost to followup. When the patient was seen in December 1978 he had an asymptomatic *E. coli 075* bacteriuria. After treatment with nitrofurantoin, this *E. coli 075* was found in the prostate. He was treated with trimethoprim-sulfamethoxazole for 60 d and his cultures showed no *E. coli 075*. After this antimicrobial was stopped his urinary tract was colonized by an *E. coli 016* and then 2 other *E. coli* serotypes. For this reason he was placed on prophylactic trimethoprim-sulfamethoxazole until January 1981 and his cultures have been sterile for gram negative organisms.

Results

From these two longitudinal studies we found that nonspecific IgG and IgA in serum were inadequate immunologic determinants of prostatic infection. Nonspecific IgA and IgG in EPS, on the other hand, were elevated during times of prostatic infection. Whether this elevation results from an increase in secretory rate or increase in production of immunoglobulin was not determined.

In patient 1 with acute bacterial prostatitis, antigen-specific IgG in both serum and prostatic fluid shows a parallel rise and fall. This observation suggests serum transudation of specific antibody into the prostate gland during acute inflammation. Simultaneously antigen-specific IgA in both serum and EPS, rises after infection, but the EPS elevation is strikingly greater in magnitude than that seen in serum and persists for months after the elevation in serum is no longer detectable (Fig. 1). This suggests local production of anti-

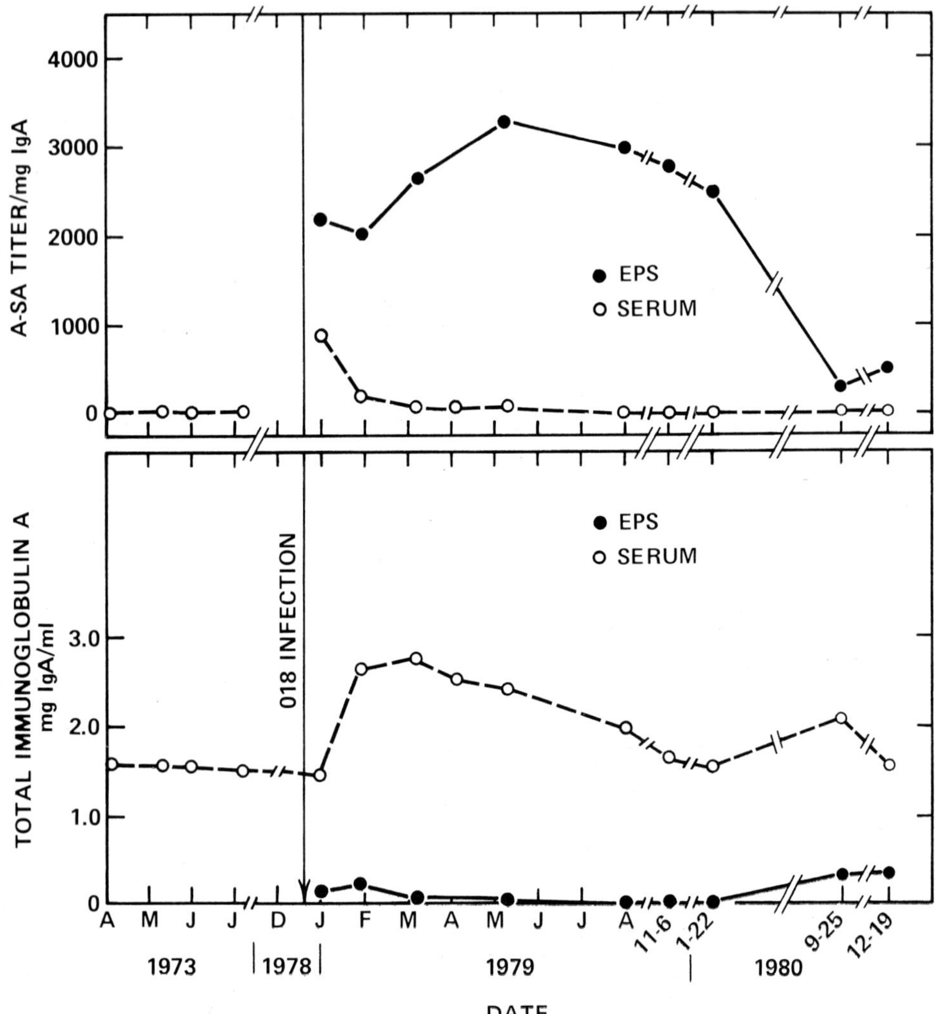

Fig. 1. A longitudinal study of the total and *E. coli 018*-specific IgA responses in the prostatic fluid and serum in patient 1 with acute bacterial prostatitis. Serum and prostatic specimens were assayed for total and *E. coli 018*-specific IgA antibodies. *E. coli 075*-specific IgA and prostatic fluid total IgA were measured in duplicate by solid-phase radioimmunoassay. Nonspecific serum total IgA was measured by radial immunodiffusion. The upper portion of the figure shows that elevation in EPS antigen-specific IgA is greater in magnitude and persists much longer than that seen in serum. Baseline levels of EPS antigen-specific antibody were reached 20 months after the acute infection. The lower portion of the figure illustrates the elevation in EPS total IgA observed following the infection, and the lack of significant elevation observed in serum total IgA. [From SHORTLIFFE et al. (3).]

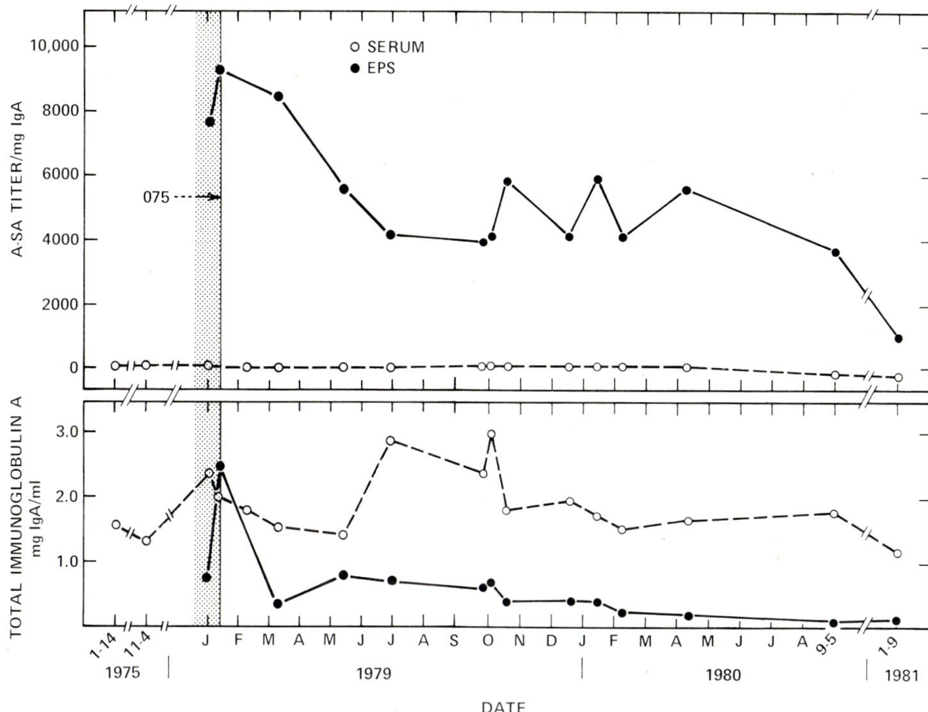

Fig. 2. A longitudinal study of the total and *E. coli 075*-specific IgA responses in serum and prostatic fluid in patient 2 with recurrent chronic bacterial prostatitis. Serum and prostatic specimens were assayed for total and *E. coli 075*-specific IgA antibodies. *E. coli 075*-specific IgA and prostatic fluid total IgA were measured in duplicate by solid-phase radioimmunoassay. Nonspecific total serum IgA was measured by radial immunodiffusion. The stippled area represents the period during which the *E. coli 075* was cultured. The upper portion of the figure illustrates the elevation in antigen-specific IgA observed up to 24 months after infection. During this period no detectable elevation in serum antigen-specific antibody occurred. The lower portion of the figure shows EPS and serum total nonspecific IgA measured during this time. [From SHORTLIFFE et al. (3).]

body within the prostate. In patient 2, infection elicits minimal elevation in serum IgG antigen-specific antibody, whereas in the prostate a significant elevation is measured. Similarly, in this second patient with chronic prostatic infection, prostatic antigen-specific IgA shows a marked elevation, whereas the systemic response is scarcely detectable (Fig. 2). This response supports evidence for the production of local immunoglobulins by the prostatic gland.

In order to test this immunoglobulin response, Dr. K. WISHNOW in the Stanford Urology Laboratories compiled two pools of enterobacteriaceae which commonly cause urinary tract infections (4). Pool 1 was composed of equal quantities of *E. coli* serotypes commonly involved in infections: 01, 02,

04, 06, 07, 018, 050, and 075; Pool 2 was composed of 6 non-*E. coli* gram negative organisms: *Klebsiella pneumoniae, Proteus mirabilis, Pseudomonas aeruginosa, Serratia marcescens, Enterobacter aerogenes,* and *Citrobacter freundi.* Males without history of urinary or prostatic infections — normal controls (22 men), males with well-documented bacterial prostatitis (12 men), and males with nonbacterial prostatitis (9 men) underwent lower tract bacterial localization as previously described. The prostatic fluid was stored and then assayed against the two antigen pools. Neither normal controls nor patients with nonbacterial prostatitis demonstrated any measureable levels of antibody against the *E. coli* or the mixed organism gram negative pools. Patients with bacterial prostatitis had a mean of 15.4 units of anti-*E. coli* IgA and 2.1 units of anti-*E. coli* IgG. Of these 12 patients with bacterial prostatitis who showed elevated antibodies against the pools, 5 of the 12 were infected with organisms or *E. coli* serotypes which were not included in our pool. Moreover, the prostatic fluid of patients with bacterial prostatitis contained more total IgA and IgG than either normal controls or patients with bacterial prostatitis.

From our studies of two patients with bacterial prostatitis we were able to demonstrate a characteristic local prostatic antibody response to bacterial infection of the prostate. These local immunologic responses were independent of serum responses. Although previous studies (3) have shown that these responses appear to be specific for the infecting *E. coli* serotype, it appears that sufficient cross-reactivity between different gram negative organisms and *E. coli* serotypes occurs that elevation of prostatic antibodies to screening enterobacteriaceal pools can be measured. Although serum responses are short-lived, local antigen-specific immunoglobulin can be detected for as long as two years after the initial infection. Local secretory immunoglobulin A appears to be the principal immunoglobulin involved in this response. From further studies involving males without history of infection and males with bacterial and nonbacterial prostatitis, it appears that the detection of antibodies against enterobacteriaceae in the prostatic fluid is diagnostic of bacterial prostatitis.

References

(1) Zollinger, W. D., J. M. Dalrymple, M. S. Artenstein: Analysis of Parameters Affecting the Solid Phase Radioimmunoassay Quantitation of Antibody to Meningococcal Antigens. J. Immunol. *177*: 1788—1797 (1976).

(2) Shortliffe, L. M. D., N. Wehner, T. A. Stamey: The Use of a Solid Phase Radioimmunoassay and Formalin-fixed Whole Bacterial Antigen in the Detection of Antigen-Specific Immunoglobulin in Prostatic Fluid. J. Clin. Invest. *67*: 790—799 (1981).

(3) Shortliffe, L. M. D., N. Wehner, T. A. Stamey: The Detection of a Local Immunoglobulin Response to Bacterial Prostatitis. J. Urol. *125*: 509—515 (1981).

(4) Wishnow, K. I., N. Wehner, T. A. Stamey: The Diagnostic Value of the Immunologic Response in Bacterial and Non-bacterial Prostatitis. J. Urol. *127*: 689—694 (1982).

Division of Urology, Stanford University School of Medicine, Stanford, Calif.
The Institute for Medical Research, Santa Clara Valley Medical Center, San Jose, Calif.

Immunological Studies in Abacterial Prostatitis

R. U. ANDERSON, S. H. MA

Introduction

Abacterial prostatitis continues to afflict many men and baffle most urologists. We lack good definitions of this disorder due to poor understanding of the pathophysiology, hence we tend to categorize most patients with pelvic/prostate complaints as suffering with *prostatitis*. Only those patients who demonstrate increased white cell proliferation in their prostatic secretion should carry the diagnosis of prostatitis, whether of bacterial or nonbacterial etiology. [DRACH et al. (1); ANDERSON and WELLER (2); SCHAEFFER et al. (3)]. By adhering to this definition of prostate gland inflammation, we can expand investigations of the nature of the disease; i.e., search for microbiologic, immunologic, neurologic, or psychologic etiologies.

In this work we sought to detect evidence of auto-antibody associated with abacterial prostatitis. We studied all male subjects referred to the urology clinic with urethral, prostate, or pelvic complaints and no apparent bacterial infection. Careful bacterial and leukocyte localization was done and then patients were screened for any evidence of a humoral auto-antibody reaction to prostate tissue using a passive hemagglutination technique.

Materials and methods

All patients were carefully questioned about their complaints. We scored (1 to 3 plus) specific symptoms to identify patterns of the syndrome. The patient voided and a urethral washout specimen (<10 mls) was collected followed by a second midstream specimen caught late in the urinary flow. After careful compression of the urethral bulb, prostate fluid was collected by gland massage: urethral compression prior to massage helped insure that no excess urine would dilute the expressed prostate secretion (EPS). The specimens were taken immediately to the laboratory for standard bacterial cultures. Fifty ml of blood was obtained from each patient by venipuncture.

Cytology: We counted cells from all specimens in an uncentrifuged condition using a Fuchs-Rosenthal counting chamber and Sternheimer-Malbin stain; a 20 microliter aliquot of prostatic secretion was diluted 1:10 with 20 microliter of Sternheimer-Malbin stain and 160 µl of diluent[1]. The cell count was performed in duplicate and the average reported. A further aliquot of prostatic secretion (10 to 20 µl) diluted in 10 to 20 ml of diluent was placed on an 8.0 ϑm millipore filter and washed with an addition 100 ml of isotonic solution. This cell concentrate was then fixed immediately in 95 per cent ethanol and stained with Papanicolaou technique. Microscopic differential analysis of these stained cells was performed in duplicate.

Humoral Antibody Screen: We used passive hemagglutination with tanned sheep red blood cells to determine the presence of any circulating anti-prostate antibody [Boyden (4); Albin (5)]. The tanned red cells were antigen coated with either the patient's own prostate secretion, pooled EPS, or pooled prostate homogenate extract, each diluted to an optimal 0.2% protein concentration. Prostate tissue was obtained from patients undergoing surgery, most commonly for benign hypertrophy and bladder outlet obstruction, and was stored at −20°C until used. This tissue from several patients was pooled, cut into small pieces and homogenized in a glass homogenizer with 2.5 ml saline per gram of tissue. The homogenate was centrifuged at 4°C for 30 minutes and the supernatant saved. The protein concentration of the pooled extract was determined by the biuret method.

Washed sheep red blood cells were treated for 30 minutes at room temperature with a 1:20,000 dilution of tannic acid. Cells tanned in this manner were washed and coated immediately, after final suspension in cold phosphate buffered saline, by mixing them with an equal volume of antigen (pooled EPS, patient's EPS, prostate homogenate) diluted to a predetermined optimal concentration of 0.2% protein. Incubation was carried out for 30 minutes at room temperature. Tanned coated cells were washed twice in 1:60 dilution (in phosphate buffered saline) of normal horse serum. Immedieately after the final washing, cells were resuspended at 2% in this diluent. All patient serum was inactivated at 56°C for 30 minutes and absorbed twice each for 30 minutes with washed sheep red blood cells. To increasing dilutions of the patient's serum, in volumes of 0.05 ml, was added 0.05 ml of a 2% suspension of the tanned coated erythrocytes. Tanned, but uncoated, sheep red blood cells acted as control cells for each serum tested. Readings were taken after 1 to 2 hours incubation at room temperature. The degrees of agglutination were graded as 4 plus to 1 plus or negative. All tubes were shaken and left overnight at 4°C and readings repeated. The titer for each series was expressed as the highest dilu-

---

[1] Isolyte-E, McGraw Laboratories, Glendale, California.

tion of serum that gave at least a 1 plus reaction. Blocking experiments with prostate antigen added to patient serum resulted in no agglutination other tissues such as kidney, intensive and bladder were also negative.

Positive Control Antiserum: Female New Zealand albino rabbits weighing 7 to 10 lb were inoculated with pooled EPS or prostate tissue emulsified with an equal volume of incomplete Freund's adjuvant. Approximately 0.1 ml of emulsion was injected intradermally into the shaved skin of the rabbit's back using five to six sites for inoculation. Inoculations were repeated weekly for 4 weeks and followed by 4 weeks of rest. Two such courses were given resulting in a total administered protein of 1.1 mg protein EPS, and 30 mg protein prostate tissue extract.

Results

We evaluated 54 males complaining of prostate or pelvic discomfort. The results of bacterial cultures from the urethral washout specimen (VB1), and mid-stream urine (VB2), and from the expressed prostatic secretion (EPS) are shown in Table 1. In many instances the colony counts from the prostatic secretion exceeded that from the urethra, but never enough to identify the bacteria as an infectious agent.

Leukocyte cell counts from the urine and EPS specimens revealed those subjects who had true prostatic inflammation, i.e., >1000 cells/mm^3 or ≥ 10 cells per high power field (Table 2). The average cell count of the patient group was 3,733 $\pm$ 858 (S.E.M.) per microliter (mm^3). Some of these patients also had high urethral cell counts but normal prostate secretion counts and were designated as urethritis patients; eleven men fell into this category. Their average VB1 cell count was 142 $\pm$ 9 per mm^3. Patients with normal cell counts in urethral, bladder and prostate specimens were assigned diagnoses based upon

Table 1: Localization of bacteria in 54 patients; average number of colonies per ml ($\pm$ S.E.M.).

Organism	Urethra	Bladder	Prostatic secretion
Staphylococcus epidermidis	2043 $\pm$ 858	483 $\pm$ 249	1019 $\pm$ 227
Alpha Streptococcus	914 $\pm$ 283	99 $\pm$ 35	3114 $\pm$ 1575
Enterococcus	2743 $\pm$ 1527	259 $\pm$ 153	2075 $\pm$ 599
Diphtheroids	466 $\pm$ 172	86 $\pm$ 32	1144 $\pm$ 308
Coliform	7 $\pm$ 3	2 $\pm$ 2	67 $\pm$ 44

Table 2. Quantified leukocyte count from the urethra (VB1) and the expressed prostatic secretion (EPS) of normal controls and patients with prostate/pelvic discomfort.

		Mean WBC per mm^3 $\pm$ S.E.M.		range
	n	VB1	EPS	
Normals	14	15 $\pm$ 4 (0– 53)	485 $\pm$ 79	(60– 987)
Patients	54	156 $\pm$ 78 (0–3243)	3,733 $\pm$ 858	(25–39354)
(A) Prostatitis	34	128 $\pm$ 73 (0–2208)	5,721 $\pm$ 247	(1080–39354)
(B) Non-Prostatitis	20	201 $\pm$ 69 (0–3243)	355 $\pm$ 62	(25– 995)

further clinical testing. There were, for example, seven patients diagnosed with interstitial cystitis, one with benign prostatic hypertrophy and bladder outlet obstruction, one with external meatal stenosis, and one subject diagnosed with a neurogenic bladder. When all investigational methods were negative, the patients were said to be suffering from *prostatodynia,* clearly a diagnosis of exclusion; ten patients fell into this category.

Fifty-four patients and fourteen normal male controls had passive hemagglutination studies performed. We also tested six normal females and none of them had detectable antibody. There was no detectable response (agglutination) to autologous or pooled homologous expressed prostatic secretion used as antigen. When testing the patient serum against prostate tissue homogenate, however, several patients had very high titers as shown in Table 3. Seventy-one per cent of the patients with elevated prostatic secretion leukocyte counts

Table 3. Humoral anti-prostate antibody titer in normal control subjects and patients.

	n	Titer mean $\pm$ S.E.M.	range	No. >1:32
Normal Controls	14	10.3 $\pm$ 4.4	<2 to 64	1 (7%)**
Nonbacterial Prostatitis	34	4,811 $\pm$ 1124*	<2 to >16,384	24 (71%)
Urethritis	6	1,580 $\pm$ 1332	<2 to 8,192	3 (50%)
Interstitial Cystitis	4	11 $\pm$ 7	<2 to 32	0
Prostatodynia	10	112 $\pm$ 67	<2 to 512	2 (20%)

 * P<0.01 as compared to normals.
** percent of subjects tested with titers >1:32.

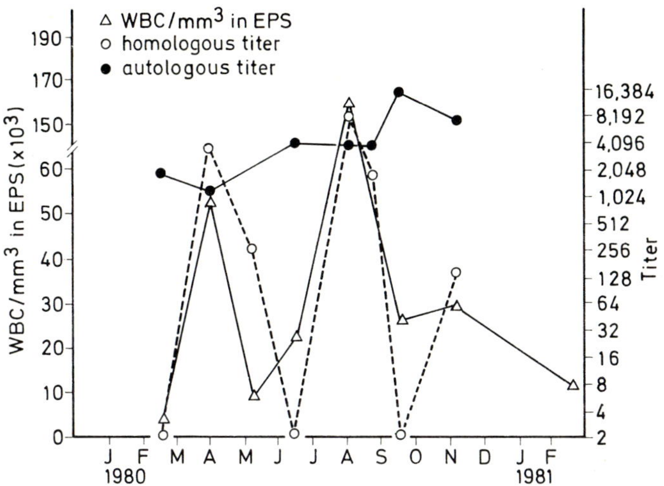

Fig. 1. Single patient longitudinal study of EPS leukocyte count, homologous and autologous humoral anti-prostate antibody titer.

(prostatitis) had serum anti-prostate antibody titers greater than 1:32. Although only six patients were found to have a pure urethritis on localization of white cells, three of them were found to possess high titers in their serum. The humoral antibody titers in patients diagnosed with non-inflammatory prostate (prostatodynia) and interstitial cystitis was uniformly low. Only one control male subject had an elevated titer (1:64).

We were able to look at auto-antibody reaction in one patient using his own prostate tissue as antigen. Fig. 1 demonstrates an example of a longitudinal study of EPS leukocyte counts, homologous and autologous humoral anti-prostate antibody titers. The titer was more consistently elevated when tested against his autologous tissue.

Discussion

Inflammatory conditions of the prostate include abacterial prostatitis — a disease poorly understood. Abacterial prostatitis has traditionally excluded gram negative and gram positive bacteria as a cause, however, when we consider possible etiologic organisms such as *Mycoplasma hominis, Ureaplasma urealyticum,* or *Chlamydia trachomatis,* aberrant forms of bacteria, these may be responsible for prostatic inflammation.

With no microbial agent isolated to define the inflammation, the diagnosis remains one of exclusion and rests upon finding increased white blood cells in the expressed prostatic secretion. It is clear that young men with no history of genitourinary disease have virtually no inflammatory cells in the urethra or prostatic secretion. SCHAEFFER et al. (3) reported a group of normal (average age 38 years) men who had only 2 WBC/high power field on a wet smear in the EPS. Our group, as well as others, have usually included healthy, but older, men as control subjects, resulting in a higher normal average number of white cells (2). It is known that men who have prostatic tissue removed because of benign hypertrophy show considerable inflammatory elements at histologic review (6). While wet smear evaluation of prostatic inflammation should suffice and is most practical for the office practice, we prefer the use of counting chambers. This obviates subjective error due to cell clumping and inadequate survey at the microscope.

It seems of paramount importance, then, to describe patients suffering from prostate/pelvic discomfort from two standpoints: 1. What microorganisms have been excluded from the EPS as etiologic agents. 2. What degree of inflammation does the patient exhibit as WBC/high power field on a fresh, wet smear or, preferably, as a quantified count in a hemacytometer?

In 1936 BARNES described a disease called toxic hyperplasia of the prostate gland (7). His concept included the idea of toxic symptoms produced by absorption of normal prostatic secretion. FLOCKS et al. (8) suggested that certain types of chronic prostatitis may have disturbances of antigen-antibody relationships as an underlying pathogenesis. It was felt that the prostate gland qualified as an organ-specific system with its own discrete antigens; that it too might suffer significant and specific tissue damage associated with immunologic mechanisms. Grimble demonstrated auto-antibody to prostate antigen in a group of patients suffering from arthritis, several of whom had Reiter's syndrome (9). He also described a small group of patients with "sub-acute prostatitis", and no further definition, as having positive sera to prostate antigen.

Auto-antibodies to prostatic tissue have been demonstrated in rabbits and, although the antibody was found to be reactive to other genital organs such as the seminal vesicles, there was no cross reactivity to organs such as liver, thyroid, vagina and serum (10). Seminal plasma, however, contained reactive antigen when checked with serum antibody from isoimmunized animals. Curiously, the accessory genital tissue of immunized rabbits did not reveal any significant histologic lesions. Guinea pigs isoimmunized with seminal vesicle homogenate did show white cell infiltration, mostly lymphocytes and plasma cells, and tubular atrophy of the glands (11).

Further studies of the normal human prostate by ABLIN et al. (12) show that at least two distinct prostatic antigens exist in addition to prostatic acid phosphatase. These antigens appear to be quite species specific. Recently one of these specific human prostate antigens was purified (13). The antigen is homogeneous, has a molecular weight of 33,000 to 34,000, and exhibits a single pI of 6.9. It is present in normal, benign hypertrophic, and malignant prostates, but absent in other human tissues.

Because of the specificity of antigens in the prostate, several investigators have looked at the levels of immunoglobulins in the prostatic secretion during a disease process. When prostatic secretion immunoglobulin levels from patients with prostatitis is compared to normals there is a significant elevation of immunoglobulins G, A, and M (14, 15). SHORTLIFFE et al. (16) report that a local prostatic immunologic response occurs specifically to a bacterial antigen and that a local IgA antigen-specific response persists for months after the serum antigen-specific response is undetectable. All previous studies failed to use lower tract bacteriologic localization techniques.

Our investigation specifically ruled out patients with bacterial prostatitis. By careful quantification of the white blood cell content in a urethral washout specimen, the bladder urine, and expressed prostatic secretion, patients were categorized as suffering from prostate inflammation, with or without simultaneous urethral inflammation.

The majority of patients with increased EPS evidence of prostate inflammation showed associated prostate antibody titers. These titers fluctuate and longitudinal studies proved to be more convincing than isolated sampling. It was interesting to note that the antibody titers may be reduced to normal in the face of persistent levels of inflammation in the EPS. Virtually all of these patients were seen many months and sometimes years after the original diagnosis of chronic prostatitis. It may require more than one inflammatory episode to raise a circulating humoral antibody.

It seems particularly relevant to evaluate with objective criteria those patients presenting with subjective and vague symptoms of prostate or pelvic pain. Quantified leukocyte testing and humoral antibody titer laboratory methods may help suggest the presence of a true chronic abacterial prostatitis. When both of these tests fall within the normal range there is increased doubt about the diagnosis and reason to pursue other investigations. Urodynamics and cystoscopy under anesthesia may reveal urethrovesical neurodysfunction or interstitial cystitis. When either the EPS leukocytes or humoral anti-prostate antibody titers are elevated, longitudinal studies and repeat testing are indicated.

This investigation does not prove that reactive antibodies are specific for the prostate, and the fact that patients with urethritis and no prostate inflammation may show elevated titers reveals its non-specific nature. Further experiments on the reactive sera using non-prostatic tissue as well as purified prostatic antigen are underway.

References

(1) DRACH, G. W., E. M. MEARES, W. R. FAIR, T. A. STAMEY: Classification of benign diseases associated with prostatic pain: Prostatitis or Prostadodynia? J. Urol. *120*: 266 (1978).

(2) ANDERSON, R. U., C. WELLER: Prostatic secretion leukocyte studies in nonbacterial prostatitis (prostatosis). J. Urol. *121*: 292 (1979).

(3) SCHAEFFER, A. J., E. F. WENDEL, J. K. DUNN, J. T. GRAYHACK: Prevalence and significance of prostatic inflammation. J. Urol. *125*: 215 (1981).

(4) BOYDEN, S. J.: The adsorption of proteins or erythrocytes treated with tannic acid and subsequent hemagglutination by antiprotein sera. J. Exp. Med. *93*: 107 (1951).

(5) ABLIN, R. J., P. BRONSON, W. A. SOANES, E. WITEBSKY: Tissue and species-specific antigens of normal human prostatic tissue. J. Immun. *104*: 1329 (1970).

(6) KOHNEN, P. W., G. W. DRACH: Patterns of inflammation in prostatic hyperplasia: a histologic and bacteriologic study. J. Urol. *121*: 755 (1979).

(7) BARNES, R. W.: Toxic hyperplasia of the prostate gland. J. Urol. *35*: 70 (1936).

(8) FLOCKS, R. H., V. C. URICH, C. A. PATEL, J. M. OPITZ: Studies on the antigenic properties of prostatic tissue, I. J. Urol. *84*: 134 (1960).

(9) GRIMBLE, A.: Auto-immunity to prostate antigen in rheumatoid disease. J. Clin. Path. *17*: 264 (1964).

(10) SHULMAN, S., C. YANTORNO, W. A. SOANES, M. J. GONDER, E. WITEBSKY: Studies on Organ Specificity, XVI. Urogenital tissues and autoantibodies. Immunology *10*: 99 (1966).

(11) ORSINI, R., S. SHULMAN: The antigens and autoantigens of the seminal vesicle. I. Immunochemical studies on guinea pig vesicular fluid. J. Exp. Med. *134*: 120 (1971).

(12) ABLIN, R. J., P. BRONSON, W. A. SOANES, E. WITEBSKY: Tissue- and species-specific antigens of normal human prostatic tissue. J. Immun. *104*: 1329 (1970).

(13) WANG, M.C., L. A. VALENZUELA, G. P. MURPHY, T. M. CHU: Purification of a human prostate specific antigen. Invest. Urol. *17*: 159 (1979).

(14) GRAY, S. P., J. BILLINGS, N. J. BLACKLOCK: Distribution of the immunoglobulins G, A and M in the prostatic fluid of patients with prostatitis. Clin. Chim. Acta *57*: 163 (1974).

(15) NISHIMURA, T., D. F. MOBLEY, C. E. CARLTON: Immunoglobulin A in split ejaculates of patients with prostatitis. Urology *9*: 136 (1977).

(16) SHORTLIFFE, L. M. D., N. WEHNER, T. A. STAMEY: The detection of a local prostatic immunologic response to bacterial prostatitis. J. Urol. *125*: 509 (1981).

*Division of Urology, Department of Surgery, Stanford University School of Medicine,
Stanford, Calif.*

Leukocyte Studies in Abacterial Prostatitis

R. U. ANDERSON

Normal prostatic secretion has very few white blood cells in it when examined microscopically. Increased numbers of leukocytes seen on a wet smear of expressed prostatic secretion has served as the basis for a clinical diagnosis of prostatic inflammation or prostatitis. It is apparent that this inflammation is sometimes caused by gram negative bacteria, possibly even gram positive bacteria, but a preponderance of patients diagnosed with prostatitis have no documentable bacterial focus in the gland. It is reported that aberrant bacterial forms such as *Ureaplasma urealyticum* and *Mycoplasma hominis* may be responsible for some cases of abacterial prostatitis (WEIDNER et al., 1980).

To pursue investigations concerning the etiology of prostatitis, be it bacteriologic, immunologic, neurologic, or psychologic, patients should have documented evidence of inflammation originating from the prostate gland. Virtually all of the previous studies of prostatitis have been hampered by inadequate definition due to poor localization of microorganisms or white blood cells in the genitourinary tract.

This investigation sought to carefully quantify the bacterial and leukocyte content of the urethra, bladder, and prostatic secretion in a group of men referred with a diagnosis of abacterial prostatitis.

Patients and methods

There were 89 male patients and 34 normal control subjects investigated. Patients were interrogated concerning their symptoms and these symptoms were subjectively graded by the examiner on a scale of 1 plus to 3 plus. Scores were given in the categories of pain, irritative voiding, and obstructive voiding symptoms.

Routine localization of bacteria and leukocytes was done according to the method described by MEARES and STAMEY (1972). The first voided specimen (VB1) represented the urethral washout and was limited to < 10 ml to eliminate a dilutional factor. A second voided midstream specimen (VB2) was collected late in the urinary flow. The prostate was massaged, after compression of the urethral bulb to express any residual urine, and the expressed prostate secretion (EPS) collected. Specimens were taken immediately to the laboratory for cultures and cytology. Bacteria were counted and reported as colonies per ml of urine and EPS. The pH of the prostatic secretion was determined using a pH meter. Cell counts were made on uncentrifuged urine after addition of Sternheimer-Malbin stain and counted in a Fuchs-Rosenthal chamber, including all cells in 1 mm^3. Duplicated sample counts were expressed as the average. EPS cell counts were made using a 20 microliter aliquot of EPS diluted 1:10 with 160 microliter of Isolyte-E[1] and 20 microliter of Isolyte-E and 20 microliter of Sternheimer-Malbin stain. Additional aliquots of EPS were prepared on a millipore filter for Papanicolaou staining. A differential cell analysis was accomplished using this stained specimen.

Results

There was no difference in the incidence of commensal organisms from the urethra and prostate between the normal control group and the patient group. In many instances the count of normal flora was higher in the EPS, but never as much as a 10-fold increase to suggest that the organisms were responsible for prostate inflammation. The mean counts of bacterial localization in the patient group are shown in Table 1.

The control group had an average urethral white blood cell count of 15/mm^3, whereas the patient group had 156/mm^3. The control group had an average EPS count of 523 WBC/mm^3, and the patient group had 4,811 WBC/mm^3. Five

Table 1: Localization of bacteria in 54 patients; average number of colonies per ml ($\pm$ S.E.M.).

Organism	Urethra	Bladder	Prostatic secretion
Staphylococcus epidermidis	2043 $\pm$ 858	483 $\pm$ 249	1019 $\pm$ 227
Alpha Streptococcus	914 $\pm$ 283	99 $\pm$ 35	3114 $\pm$ 1575
Enterococcus	2743 $\pm$ 1527	259 $\pm$ 153	2075 $\pm$ 599
Diphtheroids	466 $\pm$ 172	86 $\pm$ 32	1144 $\pm$ 308
Coliform	7 $\pm$ 3	2 $\pm$ 2	67 $\pm$ 44

---

[1] McGraw Laboratories, Glendale, California.

Table 2. Quantified leukocyte pattern in normal controls and 89 males with pelvic/prostate discomfort.

Diagnosis	n	Mean WBC/mm^3 ± S.E.M. Urethral (VB1)	Prostatic secretion
Normals	34	15 ± 4	523 ± 83
Urethritis	5	142 ± 9	600 ± 170
Abacterial Prostatitis	52	18 ± 3	5,862 ± 917
Urethroprostatitis	8	537 ± 248	2,071 ± 405
Interstitial Cystitis	7	45 ± 19	312 ± 117
Prostatodynia	17	10 ± 4	413 ± 65

patients were found to have high urethral WBC counts but normal EPS counts — these were designated as having *urethritis*. Eight patients had inflammation in both the urethra and EPS, and 52 patients had elevated WBC counts only in the EPS. Utilizing two standard deviations from the mean WBC counts of the urethra and EPS in the normal control group, we designated >50 WBC/mm^3 in the VB1 and >1000 WBC/mm^3 in the EPS as objective evidence of inflammation. This left 24 patients (27 per cent) who had no evidence of inflammation in either the urethra or EPS. The leukocyte counts by differential diagnosis are given in Table 2.

Further clinical evaluation of these patients who had no demonstrable inflammation revealed 7 of them to have significant submucosal microhemorrhages (glomerulations) in the bladder when it was dilated to capacity (up to 70 cm water pressure) under anesthesia. These patients were diagnosed with *interstitial cystitis*. There were, therefore, 17 patients relegated to the category of *prostatodynia* for lack of further definitive findings.

When patients were compared by subjective clinical scoring, the higher scoring patients had higher elevations of WBC's in the EPS ($p < 0.05$). The macrophage content of EPS averaged 13 per cent of cells from normal controls. This was increased to 26 per cent in the patient groups, but there was no correlation to the total WBC count, i.e. higher count EPS specimens did not necessarily have a higher percentage of macrophages.

Although the pH of the patient group tended to be elevated, this was not significantly different from the control group.

Discussion

An evaluation of leukocytes in the prostatic fluid is clearly an essential step in diagnosing chronic prostatitis. This should be done in conjunction with a careful localization of possible microorganisms causing inflammation. Longitudinal examinations with quantification of leukocytes in the EPS provides the clinician with convincing evidence that he is not dealing with other syndromes such as urethritis, interstitial cystitis, pelvic floor myalgia, functional voiding disorder, or prostatodynia (SEGURA et al., 1979; SIROKY et al., 1981; MEARES, 1980).

While there has been controversy concerning what constitutes a "normal" number of leukocytes in EPS, it appears that the number is something less than 10 WBC/high power field (HPF) (ANDERSON and WELLER, 1979; SCHAEFFER et al., 1981). Calculating from the leukocytes per mm³ found in our 34 normal controls, this represents an average of about 5 WBC/HPF. Two standard deviations is still 10/HPF. If all investigators used a counting chamber for WBC observations, rather than scanning a wet smear, there would be more unanimity of evaluation.

Our results suggest that patients with increased numbers of leukocytes in the EPS have higher symptom scores. It is not unusual, however, to find very symptomatic patients with normal numbers of leukocytes and these are certainly the patients who deserve further clinical evaluation. A surprisingly high percentage of these men are suffering from neurourologic dysfunction as detected by urodynamics.

References

(1) ANDERSON, R. U., C. WELLER: Prostatic secretion leukocyte studies in non-bacterial prostatitis (prostatosis). J. Urol. *121*: 292−294 (1979).
(2) MEARES, E. M. JR., T. A. STAMEY: The diagnosis and management of bacterial prostatitis. Brit. J. Urol. *44*: 175−179 (1972).
(3) MEARES, E. M. JR.: Prostatitis syndromes: New perspectives about old woes. J. Urol. *123*: 141−147 (1980).
(4) SCHAEFFER, A. J., E. F. WENDEL, J. K. DUNN, J. T. GRAYHACK: Prevalence and significance of prostatic inflammation. J. Urol. *125*: 215−219 (1981).
(5) SEGURA, J. W., J. L. OPITZ, L. F. GREENE: Prostatosis, prostatitis or pelvic floor tension myalgia? J. Urol. *121*: 168−169 (1979).
(6) SIROKY, M. B., I. GOLDSTEIN, R. J. KRANE: Functional voiding disorders in men. J. Urol. *126*: 200−204 (1981).
(7) WEIDNER, W., H. BRUNNER, W. KRAUSE: Quantitative culture of ureaplasma urealyticum in patients with chronic prostatitis or prostatosis. J. Urol. *124*: 622−625 (1980).

Centre de Cytologie, Geneva, Clinique d'Urologie, Hôpital Cantonal, Geneva

Cellular Changes in the Prostatic Massage Fluid and Prostatitis

E. JOHANNISSON, P. GRABER

The diagnosis of subclinical and chronic prostatitis is usually difficult and a matter of different opinions. Most clinicians limit the examination to a palpation of the accessory genital glands. Sometimes an additional bacteriologic culture or a microscopic examination of a wet and untreated preparation of expressed prostatic fluid is done. However, all these techniques have their limitations. The palpatory findings are often doubtful or negative particularly in the presence of a chronic prostatitis. The subjective complaints are non specific and similar to symptomes of other urogenital diseases.

As to the bacteriological cultures a negative routine bacteriological culture does not exclude an infection since a great number of microorganisms in the male reproductive system are potentially pathogenic and some of them will not be detected by routine bacteriological examination.

For the diagnosis of inflammatory condition of the male accessory glands there is certainly a need for more objective methods in the assessment of the state and function of these glands. In our hands we have found that cytological examination of the prostatic massage fluid is particularly useful.

Cytologic material from the prostate can be obtained either by massage or by fine needle aspiration. These are two methods which cannot replace each other. The fine needle aspiration of prostatic cells is suitable for cytologic diagnosis of prostatic cancer. The massage specimen is less reliable for cancer diagnosis, but more suitable for cytologic diagnosis of inflammatory condition of the prostatic gland. As a matter of fact specimen obtained by massage should be preferred to the investigation of men with suspected infection since a fine needle aspiration occasionally can cause a sepsis.

Collection of fluid

Cytologic material for detection of inflammatory changes of the prostatic gland can be obtained after a careful massage and/or squeezing of the prostate and seminal vesicles. The squeezing should be made in a systematic way and in the direction towards the center of the glands. Usually it is easier to obtain fluid if the patient has been instructed to abstain from sexual activity for 3–5 days before the examination. The expressed fluid should be collected on a clean microscopic glass slide smeared out and fixed in 95% ethanol or a spray fixative. After the massage the patient is asked to urinate and the first 10 ml of urine is collected in a glass vial, centrifuged and prepared for cytologic examination. For quantitative assessment of the latter specimen a cytocentrifugation (e. g. Cytospin, Shandon Elliot) is required. The prostatic massage specimens are stained according to the method of Papanicolaou.

Cytological findings

The cytologic material obtained by massage is representative for a major part of the glandular epithelium but due to the anatomical situation of the prostate the material is mainly from the posterior and lateral parts. The microscopic examination of the prostatic massage fluid involves certain problems due to the variety of cells that can be found in the specimens. Cells may be present not only from the prostatic epithelium but also from the seminal vesicles, ampullae ductus deferens, bulbo-urethral glands, urinary bladder and urethra. The presence of an inflammatory disease in the urogenital tract may add a variety of inflammatory changes to the expressed fluid.

The normal fluid obtained by massage or squeezing of the prostate and the seminal vesicles contains very few cells (Fig. 1). Usually some prostatic cells are found, isolated or in small clusters.

These cells are cuboidal or columnar with a round shaped nucleus about the same size as a lymphocyte. Transitional epithelial cells are also commonly found in the normal fluid. They are flat or oval not unlike parabasal squamous cells. They vary in size and measure from 10 to 30 μ in diameter. Squamous epithelial cells are often found in the prostatic massage fluid. They are in all likelihood of urethral origin. Occasionally the squamous epithelial cells have lost their nucleus and the cytoplasm has been completely cornified. This presence of such cells represents generally a skin contamination.

Inflammatory changes

To define a normal prostatic secretion in terms of inflammatory cells, all direct smears or cytocentrifuged samples containing less than 10 neutrophil leukocytes per microscopic field (× 400) are considered as normal without any

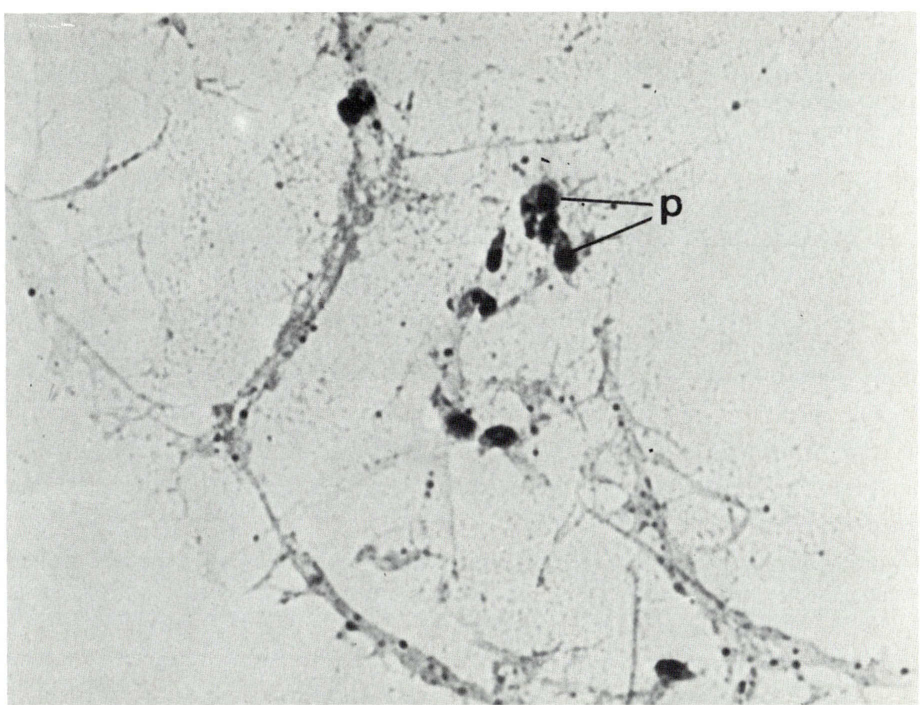

Fig. 1. Prostatic massage fluid containing less than 10 neutrophils per microscopic field representing group I. Note the presence of isolated prostatic epithelial cells (×400).

evidence of inflammation. The epithelial cells observed are well preserved and without signs of degeneration. The samples fulfilling these criteria are considered to belong to group I.

The presence of an acute or chronic inflammatory process in the prostate and/or seminal vesicles is nearly always reflected in the expressed fluid by an increased number of leukocytes and necrotic cell elements (ROMANUS, 1953; JOHANNISSON,1966; HENSCKE and MÜLLER-MARIENBURG, 1967; RIEDEL, 1973; HOFMANN, 1975; JOHANNISSON and ELIASSON, 1978; ELIASSON and JOHANNISSON, 1978). Because of the uneven distribution of the inflammatory cell elements in the direct smear it is rather difficult to state an exact number of leukocytes per microscopic field which could be consistent with a moderate or severe inflammation.

Direct smears in cyto-centrifuged urine samples obtained after massage showing clumps or secretory products containing more than 10 but less than 40 leukocytes in an average of 10 microscopic fields (×400) are considered to be consistent with inflammatory condition classified as group II (Fig. 2). Minute inflammatory changes in the prostate epithelial cells or in the transitional cells

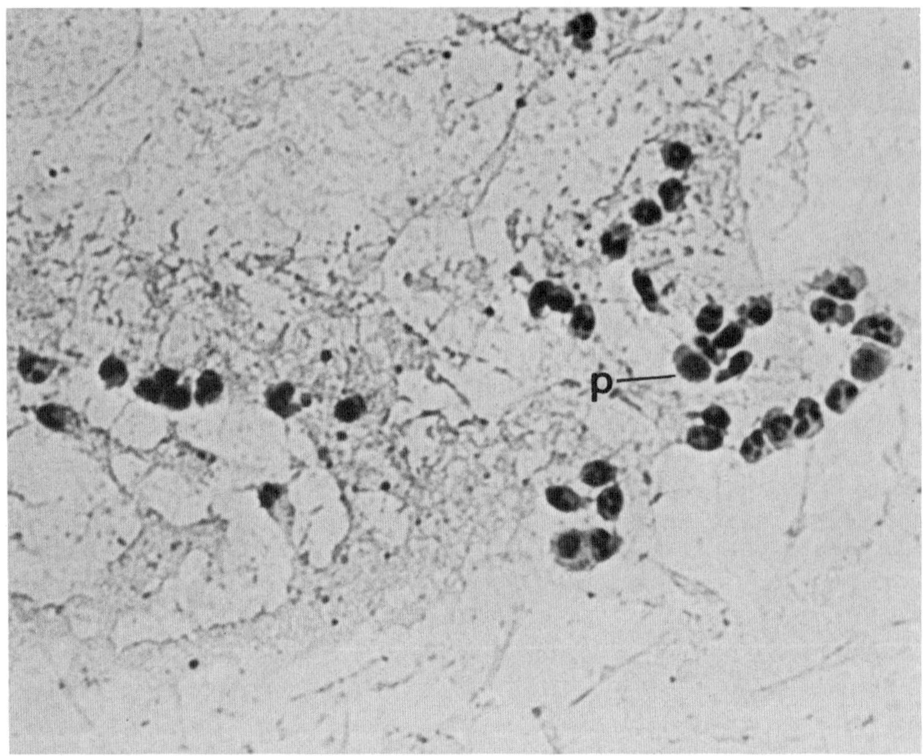

Fig. 2. Prostatic massage fluid showing a slightly increased number of neutrophils and some isolated prostatic epithelial cells (p). The presence of more than 10 but less than 40 neutrophils per microscopic field is compatible with group II ($\times$ 400).

are commonly found. The specimens belonging to this group are likely to reflect a prostatitis of infectious origin in 30% of the samples. In the other 40% the presence of inflammatory cells is likely to reflect repair or an insufficient treatment (HESSLER and GRABER, 1981).

Direct smears and cyto-centrifuged samples having more than 40 leukocytes per microscopic field and significant inflammatory changes in the epithelial cells are always reflecting an on-going inflammatory process. These specimens are classified as belonging to group III (Fig. 3). In approximately 50% a positive bacteriological finding is found (HESSLER and GRABER, 1981). In the other 50% the presence of inflammatory cells is likely to reflect an "abacterial" prostatitis, probably due to the fact that the pathogenic bacteria have not been identified in the bacteriological analyses.

Whereas the presence of neutrophil leukocytes are nearly always reflecting an acute or subacute inflammatory process the chronic inflammatory disease

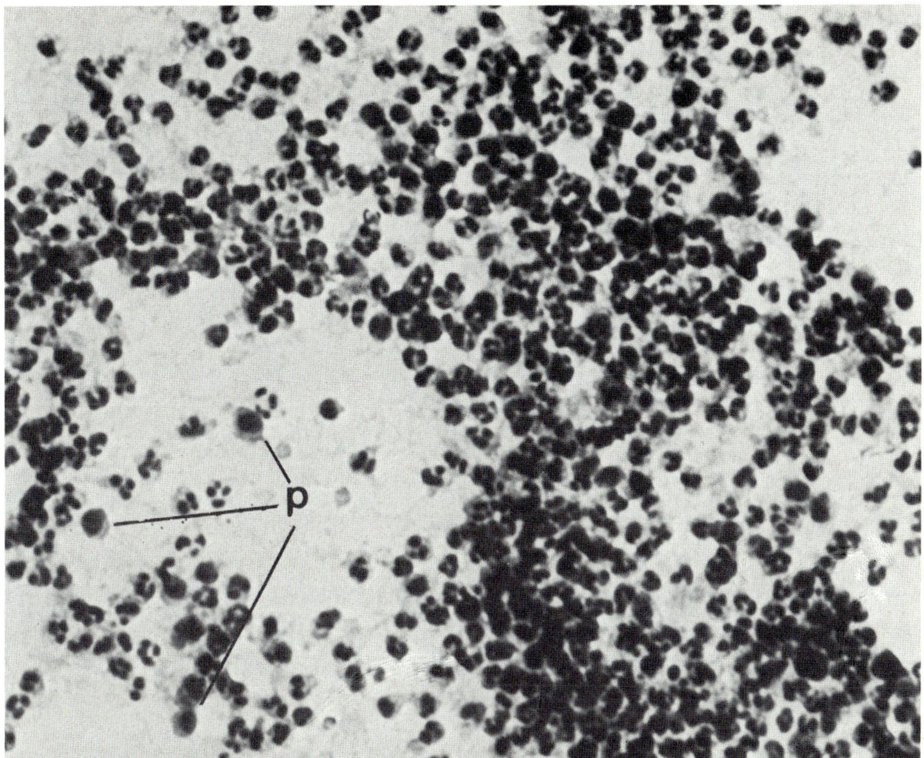

Fig. 3. Prostatic massage fluid representing a Group III inflammation. Note the presence of isolated prostatic epithelial cells (p) (×250).

reveals a different cytologic finding. The characteristic feature of the chronic inflammatory condition of the prostate and the seminal vesicles is a balance between destruction of the cellular components and repair. The cytologic findings in the prostatic massage specimen is often non specific showing only some lymphocytes and isolated prostatic epithelial cells. Usually the presence of plasma cells is significant for a chronic inflammatory process. Occasionally modifications of the epithelial cells are found corresponding to metaplasia.

Clinical application

The use of the prostate massage specimen for the diagnosis of inflammatory conditions of the male accessory genital glands is illustrated in Fig. 4. This figure refers to a study by ELIASSON and JOHANNISSON (1978) carried out in 41

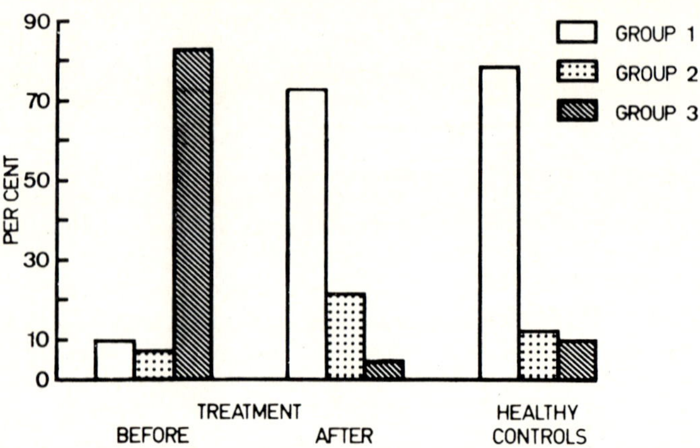

Fig. 4. Presence of inflammatory changes in the prostatic massage fluid from 41 men before and after treatment with antibacterial drugs and in healthy controls of 41 men. The prostatic massage fluid is classified in group I, II and III. [From ELIASSON and JOHANNISSON (6).]

men with palpatory and/or cytological evidence of prostatitis and in 41 healthy controls whose wives were pregnant in the first trimester. Thirty-seven or 90% of the 41 men of the study group had cytological findings compatible with inflammation before treatment. After treatment with antibacterial drugs for 6 to 16 weeks, 31 or 75.6% revealed a prostatic massage specimen free of inflammatory changes (group I). The prostatic massage specimen is therefore a useful tool not only for the diagnosis of inflammatory conditions of the male accessory glands but also for the follow-up of the treatment. Within this latter context the presence of a prostatic massage specimen of group I is an indication of a successful treatment. The administration of antibacterial drug should be discontinued except for those cases where the palpatory findings still indicate a persistent inflammation. The presence of a Group II in the prostatic massage specimen calls for further examination to clarify the type of infection. Should no specific pathogenic agents be found, the prostatic massage needs to be repeated after 4 to 5 weeks.

Persistence of Group III in the prostatic massage specimen in spite of antibacterial treatment also requires further examination. Pathogenic agents like *Chlamydia trachomatis* and *Ureaplasma urealyticum* may be responsible for the infection. Other sources of infections e.g. stenosis of urethra or prostatic stones may also be compatible with the presence of inflammatory cells in the prostatic massage specimen.

References

(1) ELIASSON, R., E. JOHANNISSON: Cytological studies of prostatic fluids from men with and without abnormal palpatory findings of the prostate. II Clinical application. Int. J. Androl. *1*: 582−588 (1978).

(2) HANSCHKE, H. S., H. M. L. MÜLLER-MARIENBURG: Cytomorphologische Befunde bei Prostatitis. Urologie *6*: 246−251 (1967).

(3) HESSLER, D., P. GRABER: La prostatite chronique. Folia chemotherapeutica. Roche *29*: 1−20 (1981).

(4) HOFMANN, N.: Fertilitätsstörungen und Chronische Entzündungen im Genitalbereich. In:. SCHIRREN, C. (ed.): Fortschritte der Andrologie; vol. 4, p. 11. Grosse Verlag, Berlin 1975.

(5) JOHANNISSON, E.: Cytologic evaluation of the prostatic massage specimen in inflammatory conditions. Proceedings of the Vth World Congress on Fertility and Sterility. Excerpta Med. Int. Congress Series *133*: 623−624 (1967).

(6) JOHANNISSON, E., R. ELIASSON: Cytological studies of prostatic fluids from men with and without abnormal palpatory findings of the prostate. I. Methodological aspects. Int. J. Androl. *1*: 202−212 (1978).

(7) RIEDEL, B.: Urologische Zytologie. Walter de Gruyter, Berlin − New York 1973.

(8) ROMANUS, E. R.: Pelvo-spondylitis ossificans in the male and genitourinary infection. Acta Med. Scan. (Suppl.) *280* (1953).

Urologische Abteilung des Krankenhauses der Barmherzigen Brüder, Wien
(Leiter: Univ.-Prof. Dr. W. Ludvik)

The Diagnostic Significance of Leucocyte Counts in Prostatic Fluid

W. LUDVIK

Inflammatory processes involving excretory glands are associated with interstitial inflammatory cell infiltration and leucocyte exudation into the glandular lumen. While controversial, it seems to be logical to regard elevated leucocyte counts in prostatic fluid samples as signs of glandular inflammation. In the literature opinions are divided on this matter (Table 1). But published studies

Table 1. Normal prostatic fluid, leucocyte count/field at high magnification: data from different sources.

CHWALLA	0
MITCHELL and VON LACKUM	5
BLUMENSAAT	10
GHORMLEY, COOK and NEEDHAM	20
O'SHAUGNESSY, PARRINO and WHITE	>50

were invariably based on unstained prostatic fluid droplets examined at high magnification, a technique which has some shortcomings.

Technique

To determine the leucocyte count in normal and abnormal prostatic fluid samples, leucocytes present in the fluid expressed from the prostate were counted in a counting chamber:

Samples were expressed by massaging the gland and collected by the patients in a graduated centrifuging tube. In the presence of urethritis patients were instructed to void beforehand.

From the collecting tube prostatic fluid was transferred to a leucocyte mixing pipette, which was filled to mark 1. Depending on the pipette size, 0.025 to

0.04 ml are required. For dilution Türk's solution was added to mark 11. Türk's solution is a 1% acetic acid containing 1 ml of a 1% aqueous Gentiana violet solution to 100 ml. It imparts a blue color to the cell nuclei so that the leucocytes can readily be distinguished from other elements present in prostatic fluid. The diluted fluid was mixed by shaking for 5 minutes and then transferred to a Fuchs-Rosenthal counting chamber. Sixteen fields were counted and multiplied by 50,000 to obtain the leucocyte count per ml.

In rare cases massaging of the prostate will not produce any fluid from the urethra even after some days of sexual abstinence. Samples will then have to be collected with the Silló-Seidl catheter for analysis (Fig. 1). The catheter is

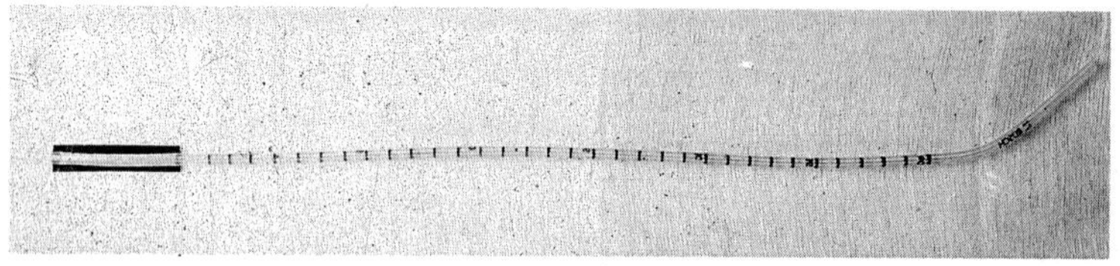

Fig. 1. Silló-Seidl catheter to obtain prostatic fluid by massage (Willy Rüsch Comp.).

introduced into the bladder and withdrawn as soon as urine appears, so that the perforated chamber comes to lie in the prostatic urethra and will be filled with prostatic fluid while the gland is massaged. The catheter technique has only been employed for preliminary studies. For routine diagnosis urinary sediments after massaging the prostate were analyzed. While this method has given satisfactory results for practical purposes, it is semiquantitative rather than quantitative in nature.

Methods

To establish the diagnostic significance of leucocyte counts in prostatitis the following examinations were done:
1. Leucocytes were counted in prostatic fluid samples from patients with chronic prostatitis diagnosed by rectal examination, clinical signs and symptoms and prostatic fluid culture;
2. leucocytes were counted in prostatic fluid samples expressed in asymptomatic subjects without any abnormalities on rectal examination and with sterile secretions;
3. leucocytes were counted in prostatic fluid samples collected before, during and after treatment for chronic prostatitis;

4. leucocytes were counted in prostatic fluid obtained from patients with adenoma of the prostate and enucleated glands were examined histologically.

Results

1. Leucocyte counts in patients with chronic prostatitis

Early results were published in 1964. A total of 44 patients with chronic prostatitis was examined. Leucocyte counts were between 300,000 and 70 million/ml. Counts below 1 million were seen in no more than 15% of cases. In the last 2 decades several thousand samples were analyzed. These confirmed the diagnostic significance of elevated leucocyte counts. We found that counts may be as high as beyond 100 million/ml. In 5% of cases counts were below 300,000/ml inspite of definitely abnormal rectal examinations and typical signs and symptoms. Secretions in these cases showed extreme depletion of lipoid droplets suggesting the presence of "burnt-out prostatitis", i.e. the end-stage of chronic prostatitis with loss of specific prostatic cell function. This condition may still be quite annoying for the patients affected. It is important to make sure that massaging systematically extends to the entire part of the prostate which is accessible to palpation. If this is not so and if areas with inflammatory lesions are missed, prostatic fluid may show a normal leucocyte count. In doubtful cases the examination should, therefore, be repeated after some days. Rarely we found prostatic fluid samples to have an extremely high lipoid droplet content and a leucocyte count in excess of 300,000/ml. This combination was seen in patients with a low ejaculate fructose level and extremely low semen volume. It is questionable in these cases whether elevated leucocyte counts reflect an inflammatory process or are secondary to inspissation of prostatic fluid.

2. Examination in normal subjects

Normal subjects were drafted men from the Austrian army. Sings or symptoms of prostatitis and abnormalities on rectal palpation were absent and secretions were sterile. Of the 45 subjects examined, 42 had leucocyte counts up to 200,000/ml. In 3 cases counts were above 300,000/ml. All of these 3 subjects had already had sexual intercourse; one had contracted gonorrhea 1 year previously. Of the subjects with leucocyte counts below 300,000/ml, 80% reported not to have had any sexual experiences yet. It should be remembered that these studies were conducted 20 years ago. They prompted us to define a leucocyte count of 300,000/ml as the upper limit of normal for prostatic fluid. This was confirmed 4 years later by Langner and Schneider, who used the same counting method.

3. Leucocyte count as a parameter for monitoring treatment

If elevated leucocyte counts in prostatic fluid reflect the presence of an inflammatory process, it is logical to expect a return to normal or at least reduction during successful treatment. This together with the elimination of the offending pathogen would seem to constitute a criterion for the successful control of the condition. That the condition is difficult to control is a well-known fact.

Between 1964 and 1966 20 patients underwent high-dose antibiotic therapy after resistance testing (Table 2). Treatment was started with fever therapy in combination with local hyperemic measures. Injections were followed by oral longterm therapy for 3 months.

Of the 20 patients thus treated, 18 were followed up at regular intervals. There were no bacteriologically verified relapses in 13 cases. In 3 patients a different pathogen was found to be present, while the same organisms persisted in 2, 1 being sensitive, the other resistant to penicillin.

Of the 13 patients, 9 responded to treatment within 4 weeks, presenting with normal prostatic fluid. Leucocyte counts continued to be normal at follow-ups

Table 2. Chronic prostatitis, highdose antibiotics.

20 patients, 1964–1966	
Na-penicillin G, 10 mio. U, b.i.d. as short infusions + Ampicillin, Oxacillin or Cephalothin, 2 g i.v., b.i.d.	28 days
Streptomycin, 0.5 g i.m. b.i.d. or Canamycin, 0.5 g i.m. b.i.d. or Colistin, 2 mio. U i.m. b.i.d.	10 days

18 patients, follow-up till 1971

Fluid culture		Leucocyte count in fluid	
		< 300,000/ml	> 300,000/ml
sterile	: 13 patients	9 patients	4 patients
new pathogen (reinfection?)	: 3 patients	– patients	3 patients
relapse	: 2 patients	– patients	2 patients

after 5 to 7 years. In 4 cases the offending pathogen was permanently eliminated, but the leucocyte counts in the prostatic fluid continued to be elevated.
There was no evidence for trichomonas, mycoplasmas or chlamydiae. We feel
that these sterile inflammations of the gland should be interpreted as a reaction
of the interstitium to secretions leaking from the glandular lumen into the
stroma. Fluid inspissation with ductal obstruction appears to play a role in this
context. Successfull elimination of the pathogen is not tantamount to a permanent cure of the inflammatory process. Its persistence can be demonstrated by
determining the leucocyte count.

4. Correlation of prostatic fluid leucocyte counts and histology

To shed light on the pathognomonic role of elevated leucocyte counts in
prostatic fluid we examined 85 patients with prostatic adenomas. Only patients
who had never had an indwelling catheter were eligible. They were aged between 53 and 76 years (mean age, 65 years).

Prostatic fluid was collected as usual pre-operatively and leucocytes were
counted using the counting chamber method. Part of the sample was collected
in a sterile test tube containing broth for cultures and resistance tests.

Prostates were removed along a suprapubic approach, superficially coagu-
lated at 4 sites by cauterization and incised with a sterile knife. From the cut
surfaces prostatic fluid was sampled with a rod-mounted swab for bacteriology.
Resected specimens were examined histologically for the presence of inflammatory infiltrations.

Leucocyte counts in the prostatic fluid expressed preoperatively were above
300,000/ml in 82 cases. Counts below this level were only present in 3 patients
(Table 3). Of the 82 patients, 31 had pathogens, 51 had sterile fluids including
the 3 with normal leucocyte counts. Patients at that time were not examined for
the presence of mycoplasmas, chlamydiae and trichomonas. Histological analysis of the enucleated glands showed inflammatory infiltrates to be present in 73
of the 82 patients with above-normal leucocyte counts. These consisted of focal
periductal lymphocyte accumulation and leucocyte-containing exudates in the
ductal lumen. As the histological examination was part of the routine assessment of the resected specimen, only a portion of the gland was screened. This
should be remembered in the 9 cases in which signs of inflammation were
absent in the sections evaluated. The 3 patients with normal prostatic fluid
samples expectedly failed to show signs of inflammation in the slices examined.
The fluid obtained from the enucleated gland and the pre-operative samples
were sterile. From the 73 specimens with inflammatory infiltrates pathogenic
organisms were cultured in 21 cases, while the fluid was found to be sterile in

Table 3. Prostatic adenoma in 85 cases.

Prostatic fluid samples expressed pre-operatively

Leucocyte count/ml	Culture	
	pathogens	sterile
> 300,000: 82 patients	31 patients	51 patients
< 300,000: 3 patients	−	3 patients

Resected specimens

Histology		Culture	
		pathogens	sterile
inflammatory infiltrates:	73 patients	21 patients	52 patients
no inflammatory infiltrate:	9 patients	3 patients	6 patients
no inflammatory infiltrate:	3 patients	− patients	3 patients

52. Of the 9 patients who showed elevated leucocyte counts but no histological evidence of inflammation, 3 were carriers of pathogens which were grown in cultures of adenoma smears and expressed prostatic fluid. Of the 6 patients with sterile smears, 2 had pathogens in the fluid sample expressed pre-operatively. This supports the assumption that closer inspection of the resected specimens would have established the presence of inflammatory lesions.

Elevated leucocyte counts in prostatic fluid samples obtained by expression appear to be consistently correlated with the presence of inflammatory infiltrates in enucleated adenomatous glands. Histological evidence of inflammatory infiltrates in cases with sterile cultures of fluid obtained from cut surfaces supports the existence of abacterial prostatitis.

Conclusion

The results presented have convinced us that the leucocyte count in prostatic fluid is a pathognomonic factor. We believe that an elevation of the leucocyte count beyond 300,000/ml reflects the exudative component of an inflammatory process.

References

(1) BLUMENSAAT, C.: Die entzündlichen Erkrankungen der Prostata. Enke, Stuttgart 1961.

(2) CHWALLA, R.: Pathophysiologie der Prostata und der Prostatahypertrophie. Urol. int. *3*: 273−296 (1956).

(3) FLAMM, H., K. S. SACHDEV, W. LUDVIK, H. JANISCH, G. NIEBAUER: Urogenitalinfektionen durch PPLO (Mykoplasmen), I. Mitteilung. Wien. klin. Wschr. *79*: 161−164 (1967).

(4) GHORMLEY, K. O., E. N. COOK, G. M. NEEDHAM: Chronic prostatitis, a urologic quandary. J. Amer. med. Ass. *153*: 915−918 (1953).

(5) LANGNER, D., H.-J. SCHNEIDER: Die Therapie der chronischen Adnexitis des Mannes. Z. Urol. *61*: 795−800 (1968).

(6) LUDVIK, W.: Zur Diagnostik der chronischen Prostatitis. Dtsch. med. Wschr. *89*: 2366−2369 (1964).

(7) LUDVIK, W.: Neue Wege der Diagnostik und Therapie der chronischen Prostatitis. Acta chir. Acad. Sci. hung. *5*: 319−332 (1964).

(8) LUDVIK, W.: Zur Therapie der Infertilität bei Pyospermie. Wien. med. Wschr. *114*: 825−827 (1964).

(9) LUDVIK, W., K. S. SACHDEV, H. FLAMM: Urogenitalinfektionen durch PPLO (Mykoplasmen), II. Mitteilung: PPLO bei chronischer Prostatitis und Urethritis. Wien. klin. Wschr. *79*: 180−183 (1967).

(10) LUDVIK, W.: Untersuchungen zur Bewertung der Leukozytenvermehrung und des Keimnachweises im Prostatasekret. Z. Urol. *64*: 613−615 (1971).

(11) MITCHELL, J., W. H. V. LACKUM: Chronic prostatitis and vesiculitis, physical and microscopic data. Brit. J. Urol. *1*: 277−284 (1929).

(12) O'SHAUGNESSY, E. J., P. S. PARRINO, J. D. WHITE: Chronic prostatitis − fact or fiction? J. Amer. med. Ass. *160*: 540−542 (1956).

(13) SILLÓ-SEIDL, G.: Analytischer Katheter für die Untersuchung von Prostata- bzw. Samenbläschenexprimat. Urologe *2*: 419−420 (1963).

Urologische Klinik, Zytologisches Labor im Zentrum für Pathologie,
Klinikum der Justus-Liebig-Universität Gießen

Cytological Analysis of Urine After Prostatic Massage (VB3) — A New Technique for a Discriminating Diagnosis of Prostatitis

W. Weidner, H. Ebner

Introduction

Classification of prostatitis according to Drach, Meares, Fair and Stamey (1978) depends upon the analysis of prostatic fluid for leucocytes. High and low numbers of these cells are well established for discrimination between prostatitis and prostatodynia.

There is much debate regarding the number of leucocytes in a smear of prostatic secretions considered to be pathologic. Even the authors mentioned above suppose different numbers to be decisive — Meares and Stamey consider 10, Drach and Fair 20 leucocytes to be the critical cytological value for diagnosis of prostatitis. These data were obtained using the high power field without exact specification of magnification.

Considering this problem, Anderson and Weller (1979) have developed a new quantitative technique for cytological analysis of EPS[1]. They consider as normal value < 1000 leucocytes/mm^3 using a Fuchs-Rosenthal chamber for determination. The authors emphasize the practicability of the method, if prostatic fluid is obtained in sufficient amounts.

This is an our opinion the uncertain aspect of this method: does enough prostatic fluid really exist at the orificium externum urethrae for common microbiological examination, special microbiological examination for mycoplasmas and chlamydiae and quantitative cytological analysis? What about the "dry prostate" in recurrent prostatitis, where insufficient amounts of EPS are obtainable due to chronic obturation of the ducts? What about the findings of Schnierstein (1965), who has demonstrated in 41 percent of men with prostatodynia the impossibility to get enough secretion for analysis?

---

[1] Expressed prostatic secretions.

Considering these questions our study group has developed a new technique for the determination of leucocytes in urine after prostatic massage, which corresponds closely to the microbiological analysis according to MEARES and STAMEY (1968). The main idea behind this technique is the following: Prostatic massage induces outlet of pyuric secretions from the prostatic ducts into the posterior urethra. The urine after prostatic massage must wash all leucocytes out of the pars prostatica urethrae. Comparing identical aliquots of urine before and after P. M.[1], increased leucocyte numbers must indicate the existence of prostatitis, provided the bladder urine does not contain leucocytes, i.e. urethritis and cystitis must be excluded.

Patients, methods

Patients: 282 men (age $\bar{x}$ 39 years, 18−70) attending Giessen "Prostatitis" out-patient department and 65 healthy controls (age $\bar{x}$ 37 years, 18−60) were examined.

Diagnostic procedures: Diagnostic procedures included case history, somatic examination, uroflowmetric and x-ray studies of the upper urinary tract (WEIDNER, 1984). Central point of diagnostic procedure was the four-specimen technique according to MEARES and STAMEY (1968). This technique included quantitative determination of common bacteria and mycoplasmas in all speci-mens. Furthermore urethral swabs after P. M. were analyzed for *Chlamydia trachomatis* and *Neisseria gonorrhoeae.* All data of microbiological analysis were published in detail (WEIDNER et al., 1978, 1980, 1982; BRUNNER et al., 1983).

Cytological analysis of urine specimens: 3 ml of midstream urine (VB2) and urine after prostatic massage (VB3) were analyzed. For this purpose two ali-quots were taken from identical amounts (about ~ 10 ml) of the two urine specimens. After cytocentrifugation the whole material was given on a slide. Papanicolaou stain followed. The technique is demonstrated in Fig. 1.

The cytological analysis was performed for urothelial cells, prostatic epithelia, cells of the seminal vesicles and of the urethra. The leucocyte popula-tion was analyzed for polymorphonuclear granulocytes, macrophages as well as for lymphocytes and plasma cells. Erythrocytes were documented too.

Because of their characteristic cytological appearance, only the number of granulocytes was considered for determination of inflammation. The semi-quantitative determination was performed using 5 view fields (400 ×: $40 \times 8 \times 1.25$ − objective 40, view field 18). The view field with the highest

---

[1] Prostatic massage.

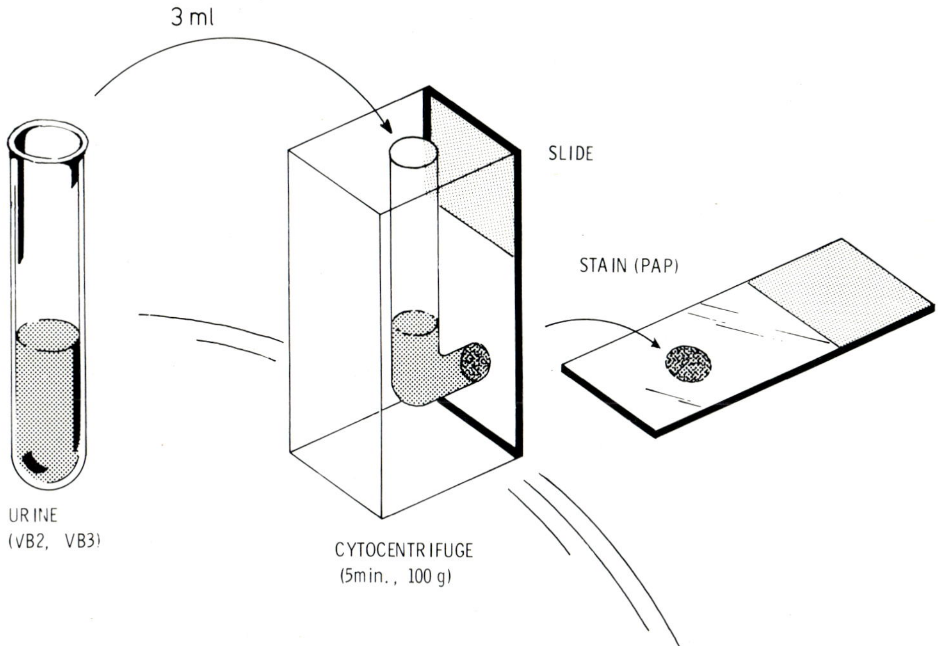

Fig. 1. Scheme of cytological technique.

amount of granulocytes was decisive for our analysis. We subdivided as follows: none, −2, −4, −10, −20 and more granulocytes.

Comparison of leucocytes in EPS and cytological analysis of VB3: In 73
healthy controls, men with prostatitis and men with prostatodynia, numbers of
leucocytes in EPS (HPF/1000×) and numbers of granulocytes in VB3 (400×)
were compared.

Results

Controls: In 65 healthy men microbiological analysis gave no evidence for
diagnosis of prostatitis. In these men, the number of granulocytes in VB2 did
not exceed 2 per view field. Analysis of VB3 demonstrated in 48 men none, in
17 up to 2 granulocytes per view field (Table 1). Even in 7 cases with positive
chlamydiae culture findings in urethral swabs after P.M., number of granulocytes was not higher.

Urethritis, epididymitis, "balanitis": In 7 men suffering from urethritis,
granulocytes were already increased (>2) in VB2. The VB3 aliquot revealed
equally high numbers of granulocytes. Cases with balanitis (n=4) and epididymitis with concomitant urethritis (n=13) showed an identical distribution of

Table 1. Analysis of numbers of granulocytes in VB3 (400×) in 65 healthy men and 233 patients suffering from symptoms of prostatitis. CBP: chronic bacterial prostatitis; UP: ureaplasma-associated prostatitis; SP: specific prostatitis; C+: positive isolation of C. trachomatis.

Granulocytes in VB3 (400×)	Healthy men (n = 65)	CBP (n = 22)	UP (n = 22)	SP.P (n = 4)	C+ (n = 43)	Without significant (n = 142) microbiol. findings
no	48	–	–	–	11	61
– 2	17^1	–	–	–	6	44
– 4	–	4^2	6^3	–	6	17
–10	–	8^2	12	3	13	14
–20	–	5	2^3	–	3	4
>20	–	5	$2^{3/3}$	1	4	2

[1] positive isolation of C.trachomatis in 7 men.
[2] mixed infection with U.urealyticum in 2 cases.
[3] additional positive isolation of C.trachomatis in 4 patients.

granulocytes in VB2 and VB3. In these cases increased numbers of granulocytes (>2) in VB3 did not differ from VB2.

Upper urinary tract infection: In 21 men with significant bacteriuria *(E.coli, S.faecalis)* both specimens showed typical pyuria.

Prostatic abscess: In 2 men prostatic abscess was evident. Bacteriologic studies revealed classic mid-stream bacteriuria *(E.coli)*. After cautious rectal palpation, VB3 demonstrated pyuria (Fig. 2).

Prostatitis

For the remainder of our examination only patients were considered for cytological diagnosis of prostatitis, in whom numbers of granulocytes in VB2 did not exceed 2 granulocytes per view field (400×). Thus patients with urethritis, balanitis, epididymitis, upper urinary tract infection and prostatic abscess could be excluded. According to these criteria 233 men remained in the study.

Increased numbers of granulocytes in VB3: Table 1 demonstrates the granulocyte score in VB3 of these remaining 233 men. 122/233 men (52.4%) had an identically low number of granulocytes as the healthy controls; 72 of the men had no granulocytes, in 50 a maximum of 2 granulocytes was demonstrable. In 111 men (47.6%) numbers of granulocytes were above 2.

Comparison of leucocyte numbers in VB3 and EPS: Table 2 demonstrates the comparison of granulocyte numbers in VB3 (400×) and the number of leucocytes in a fresh smear of EPS (1000×). VB3 specimens with granulocyte numbers up to 2 per view field showed in all cases low numbers of leucocytes in EPS

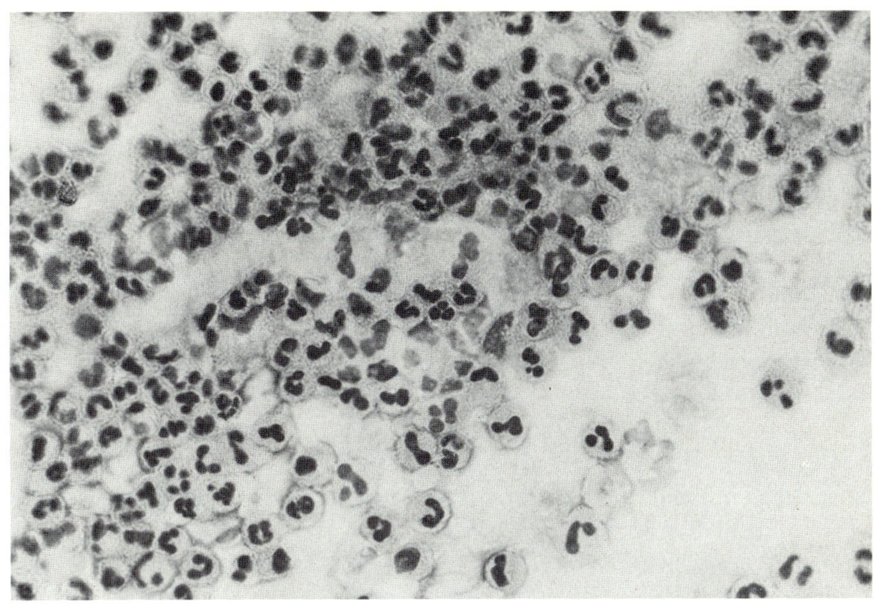

Fig. 2. Pyuria in VB3 (400×) in a patient with prostatic abscess (PAP-stain).

(<10). Significantly increased numbers of granulocytes in VB3 (≥10) were accompanied with one exception with high numbers of leucocytes in EPS (≥10). The EPS of the mentioned one patient demonstrated 5 leucocytes/HPF. Only the range from 2−4 granulocytes in VB3, i.e. a twofold increase as compared to the controls, did not correlate to the EPS score in all cases.

Granulocyte score in VB3 and microbiological classification: In 22 men (9.4%) chronic bacterial prostatitis was established. In 19 men significant numbers of gramnegative bacteria (n = 12) and enterococci (n = 7) were evident in the four-specimen technique (10 fold higher numbers of bacteria in EPS and

Table 2. Comparison of numbers of granulocytes in VB3 (400×) with numbers of leucocytes in EPS (HPF, 1000×) (n = 73).

Granulocytes in VB3 (400×)	Leucocytes in EPS (HPF, 1000×)		
	<10	10−20	>20
no − 2	46	−	−
− 4	3	4	−
−10	−	10	3
≥20	1	2	4

VB3 than in VB1 and VB2). In 3 patients identically significant numbers of other grampositive bacteria (*S.aureus* 1×, *S.haemolyticus* group A 2×) were determined. Two of these patients showed a mixed infection with significant numbers of *U.urealyticum*. As demonstrated in Table 1, numbers of granulocytes exceeded in every case the range of the healthy controls.

Ureaplasma-associated prostatitis: In 22 men (9.4%) ureaplasma-associated prostatitis with typical histograms using the 4-specimen method (VB1/VB2 $< 10^3$ cfu/ml; VB3 $\geq 10^3$ cfu/ml; EPS $\geq 10^4$ cfu/ml) was diagnosed microbiologically. All VB3 specimens revealed a minimum of 4 granulocytes; 16/22 men had even higher numbers of granulocytes (see Table 1). In 4 cases, *Chlamydia trachomatis* culture was positive too.

Specific prostatitis: In 4 men, prostatitis was established due to positive culture of *M.tuberculosis* (1×) and positive culture of *T.vaginalis* (3×). Extremely high numbers of granulocytes were evident in all cases.

Prostatitis and positive cultural findings of C.trachomatis: The significance of positive cultural findings of *C. trachomatis* in urethral swabs is discussed in detail in this book (KRAUSS et al., 1983). In 43/233 men isolation was positive, but in only 26 of the patients (11.2%) granulocyte numbers were increased. In 17 men positive cultural findings of *C. trachomatis* seemed to be commensals, because numbers of granulocytes did not differ from healthy controls.

Prostatitis without significant microbiological findings: In 37 men increased granulocytal findings were obvious without positive microbiology. In 12 of these cases recurrent non-gonococcal or gonococcal urethritis was evident in medical history, although neither urethral discharge nor high leucocyte numbers in VB1 provided evidence for actual urethritis. In further 16 cases severe radiologic inflammatory lesions in the posterior urethra, i.e. extravasation, urethritis posterior, retrograde filling of the prostatic ducts demonstrated older inflammatory alterations in the gland.

Only in 9 patients increased numbers of granulocytes could not be explained (Table 3).

Table 3. Granulocyte score (VB3/400×) in 37 men suffering from prostatitis without significant microbiological findings. NGU: nongonococcal urethritis; GU: gonococcal urethritis.

Granulocytes in VB3 (400×)	Prostatitis without significant microbiological findings		
	post NGU post GU	Urethritis posterior	not explainable
− 4	3	8	6
−10	5	8	1
−20	3	−	1
>20	1	−	1

Cytological appearance of leucocytes in VB3: It is typical for inflammatory urine cytology in prostatitis to reveal no or very few granulocytes in VB2 and many granulocytes in VB3 (Fig. 3). In many cases also macrophages were

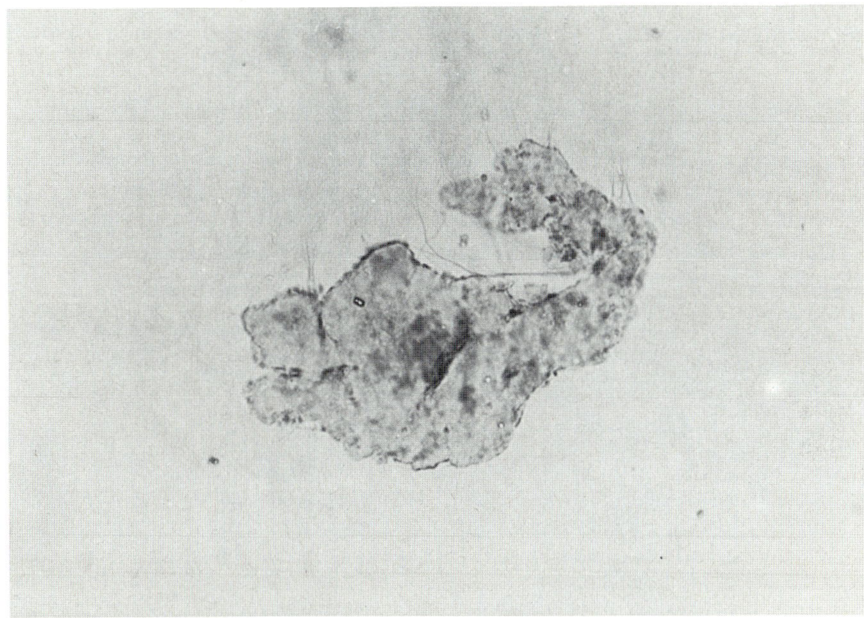

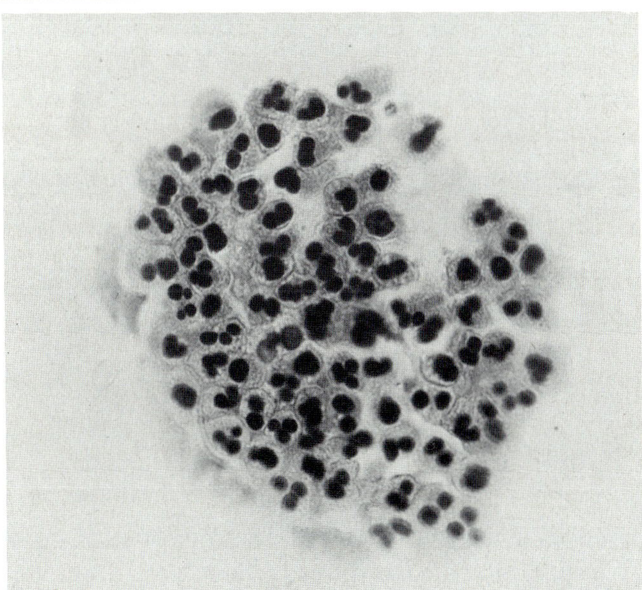

Fig. 3. Typical picture of VB2 *(above)* and VB3 *(below)* specimens with evidence of granulocytes in VB3 in a patient with chronic bacterial prostatitis (400× PAP-stain).

visible, but the occurrence of these cells did not depend upon the microbiological classification. Most of these cells could be identified due to their vacuolar degeneration (Fig. 4), moreover macrophages with evidence of inclusions in some cases (Fig. 5) were detectable. In specific prostatitis due to *Mycobacterium tuberculosis,* the cytological picture of VB3 was complicated by the evidence of "epitheloid"-cells in clusters (Fig. 6). Lymphocytes occurred very seldom, typically this finding was obvious in cases of chronic bacterial prostatitis in the follow-up after antibiotic therapy.

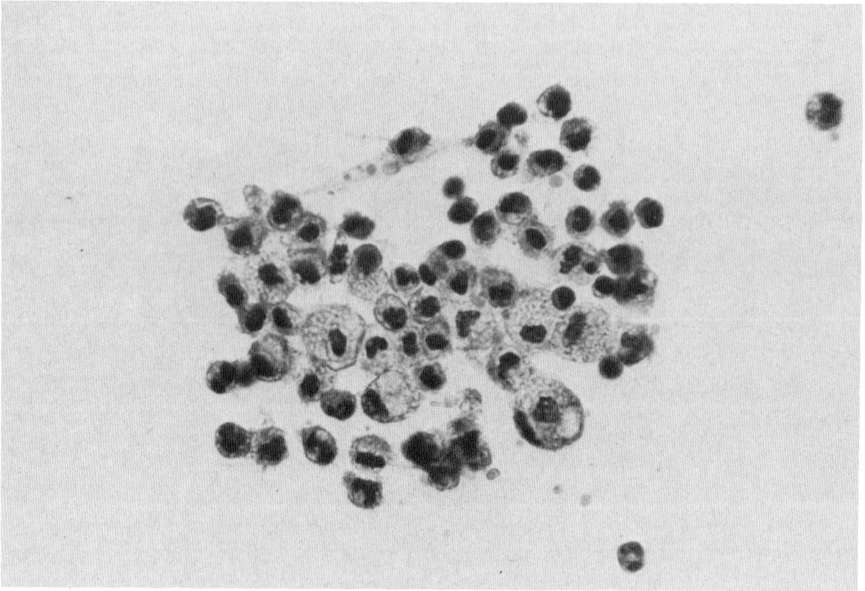

Fig. 4. Evidence of granulocytes and macrophages in a VB3 specimen of a patient with ureaplasma-associated prostatitis (400 × PAP-stain).

Discussion

Cytological analysis of urine after prostatic massage (VB3) for granulocytes provides an excellent insight into the cellular inflammatory composition of prostatic secretions.

In healthy controls, analysis of VB3 reveals in most cases no or only a few granulocytes, a result, which correlates excellently with recent results in cytological analysis of EPS (SCHAEFFER et al., 1981). As evident in this study, these authors have found slightly increased leucocyte numbers only in patients

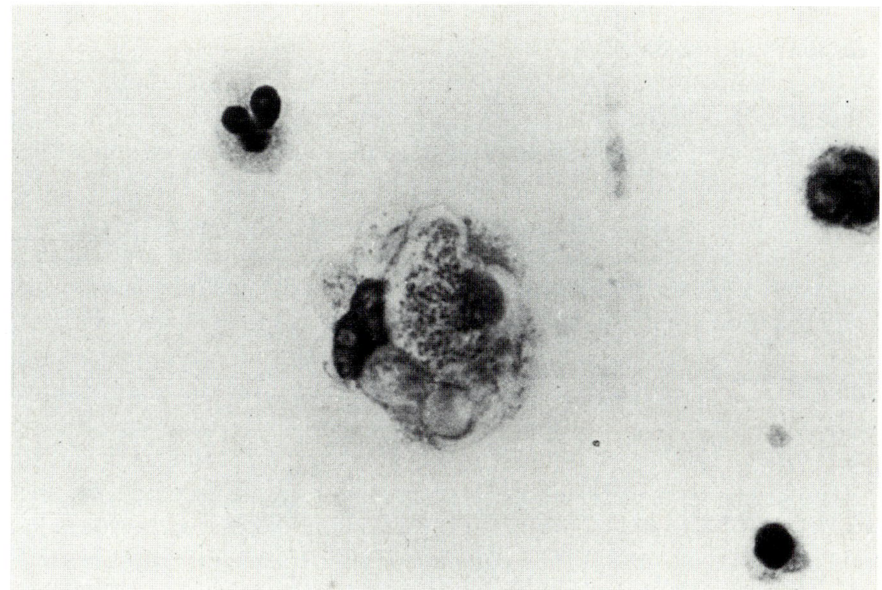

Fig. 5. Macrophages with inclusions in VB3 (1000× PAP-stain) of a patient with prostatitis and positive chlamydial findings.

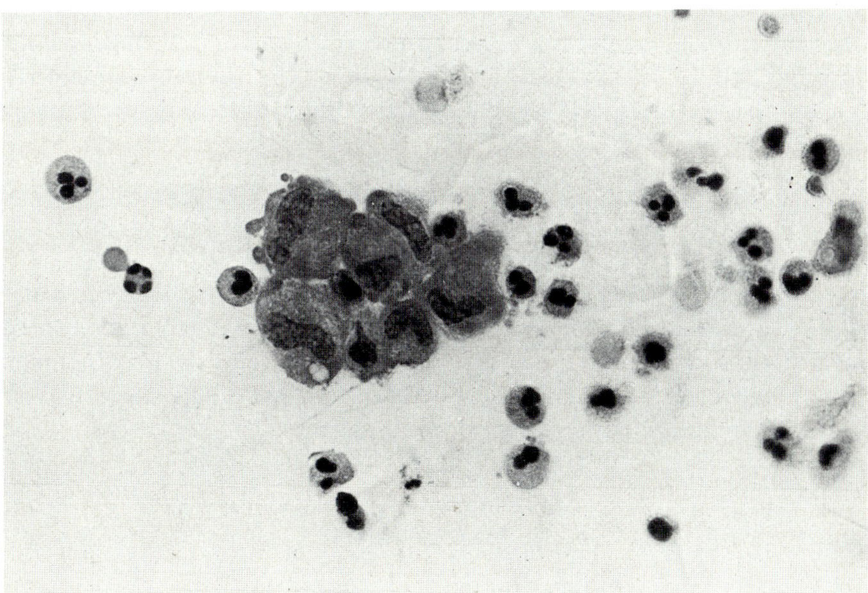

Fig. 6. "Epitheloid-similar" cells (macrophages) and granulocytes in VB3 (400× PAP-stain) in a patient with specific prostatitis (M. tuberculosis).

with bladder outlet obstruction and not in other healthy men, a finding, which corresponds to our data.

In cases of prostatitis, pyuric prostatic secretions extrudes into the posterior urethra after prostatic massage. If the total amount of cells is determined after cytocentrifugation of identical aliquots of urine before and after prostatic massage, the granulocytes must originate from the prostatic gland, if the VB2 specimen has been found to be free of leucocytes.

Performing the four-specimen method, the urine volumes are varying between 5 and 10 ml in normal cases. This makes possible a 2-fold dilution-factor, i.e. the method itself might influence the range of granulocytes. In cases of positive microbiological findings, most specimens of VB3 demonstrate a minimum of 10 granulocytes, i.e. a 5-fold increase in the number of granulocytes as compared to the normal controls. This conclusion does not only apply to cases of chronic bacterial and specific infection, but is similar in cases with ureaplasma-associated prostatitis. The cases with positive culture findings of *C.trachomatis* represent a special problem and are discussed elsewhere in this book (KRAUSS et al., 1983). The comparison of the granulocyte counts in VB3 with the cytological analysis of smears of EPS is in accordance with findings in cases in which granulocyte numbers in VB3 are equal to or exceed 10 granulocytes, whereas in cases in which the number of granulocytes does not exceed 4, there is less concordance with the EPS analysis.

Morphologically the leucocyte composition of VB3 demonstrates the inflammatory situation by the occurrence of granulocytes and macrophages as others have described (ANDERSON and WELLER, 1979). Further investigations are necessary to confirm special leucocyte-reactions in different forms of prostatitis.

Conclusion

In conclusion, the data demonstrate the number of granulocytes in VB3, to be a relevant cellular parameter of prostatitis for diagnosis in chronic bacterial, ureaplasma-associated and specific forms of the disease. If the midstream urine is free of leucocytes, then ≥ 4 granulocytes in VB3 are highly suggestive while ≥ 10 granulocytes are pathognomonic for prostatitis.

Acknowledgement

With thanks for technical assistance to Miss E. RODENBERG.

References

(1) ANDERSON, R. U., CH. WELLER: Prostatic secretion leucocyte studies in non-bacterial prostatitis (prostatosis). J. Urol. *121*: 292 (1979).

(2) BRUNNER, H., W. WEIDNER, H. G. SCHIEFER: Studies on the role of Ureaplasma urealyticum and Mycoplasma hominis in prostatitis. J. Infect. Dis. *147*: 807 (1983).

(3) DRACH, G. W., E. M. MEARES, W. R. FAIR, T. A. STAMEY: Classification of benign diseases associated with prostatic pain: prostatitis or prostatodynia? (Letter to the editor.) J. Urol. *120*: 266 (1978).

(4) KRAUSS, H., H. G. SCHIEFER, W. WEIDNER, M. ARENS, H. EBNER: Significance of Chlamydia trachomatis in "abacterial" prostatitis. Zbl. Bakt *254*: 545 (1983).

(5) MEARES, E. M., T. A. STAMEY: Bacteriologic localization patterns in bacterial prostatitis and urethritis. Invest. Urol. *5*: 492 (1968).

(6) SCHAEFFER, A. J., E. F. WENDEL, J. K. DUNN, J. T. GRAYHACK: Prevalence and significance of prostatic inflammation. J. Urol. *125*: 215 (1981).

(7) SCHNIERSTEIN, J.: Fehler und Grenzen der Prostatitis-Diagnostik. Urologe A *4*: 170 (1965).

(8) WEIDNER, W., H. BRUNNER, W. KRAUSE, C. F. ROTHAUGE: Zur Bedeutung von Ureaplasma urealyticum bei unspezifischer Prostata-Urethritis. Dtsch. med. Wschr. *103*: 465 (1978).

(9) WEIDNER, W., H. BRUNNER, W. KRAUSE: Quantitative culture of Ureaplasma urealyticum in patients with chronic prostatitis or prostatosis. J. Urol. *124*: 622 (1980).

(10) WEIDNER, W., H. G. SCHIEFER, H. KRAUSS, J. ENGSTFELD: Untersuchungen zur Ätiologie der nicht-gonorrhoischen Urethritis. Dtsch. med. Wschr. *107*: 1227 (1982).

(11) WEIDNER, W.: Moderne Prostatitisdiagnostik. In: SCHMIEDT, E., J. ALTWEIN, H. W. BAUER (eds.): Fortschritte der klinischen und experimentellen Urologie. Zuckschwerdt, München−Bern−Wien 1984.

Andrologische Abteilung der Universitäts-Hautklinik Düsseldorf (Direktor: Prof. Dr. G. Plewig)
Institut für Chemotherapie der Bayer AG, Wuppertal

Clinical, Spermatological, and Microbiological Findings in Patients with Fertility Disorders and Chronic Prostatitis

N. HOFMANN, H. BRUNNER, G. HAMMER, O. KURZ

Chronic prostatitis is found more frequently during fertility-consultations than one would expect from case-histories and clinical symptoms. In the early 1970's, we diagnosed chronic prostatitis in 14.3% of the patients in a southern German fertility clinic (HOFMANN, 1975), primarily oriented to medium and smaller cities, and in 7.4% of the cases in the early 1980's in a western German fertility clinic oriented to larger cities. The disease was generally characterized as a *"silent genital infection"*. The patients usually did not complain of present or past symptoms; the primary motive for consultation was the desire to have children (HOFMANN and WILSCH, 1973; HOFMANN, 1975). In addition, clinical findings wcrc usually not significant. Chronic prostatitis was discovered during the routine fertility examination.

Diagnosis of chronic prostatitis in fertility patients was established on the basis of the following investigations:

1. Semen analysis: increased number of leucocytes.
2. Microbiological semen analysis: *Escherichia coli, Streptococcus faecalis, Proteus mirabilis, Klebsiella pneumoniae, Neisseria gonorrhoeae, Ureaplasma urealyticum.*
3. VB1, VB2, EPS and VB3 (for definition see BRUNNER et al., page 63—73):
   a) threads in VB1 and VB3,
   b) increased numbers of leucocytes in VB1, EPS and VB3,
   c) microbiological findings in these samples, completed by investigations for *Chlamydia trachomatis* at the time of consultation.

In semen, the number of leucocytes was determined as follows:

1. counting of spermatozoa and round cells (spermatids, epithelial cells and leucocytes) in a counting chamber,
2. percent-calculation of leucocytes in Papanicolaou-stained semen smears, adjusted to 200 spermatozoa,
3. expression after this calculation as million leucocytes per ml of semen.

We established the threshold value of leucocytes in semen at 1 million/ml of semen, whereby it must be mentioned that in 20% of the patients with leucocyte counts of 1 million/ml of semen, no infectious agent could be detected. The interpretation in these cases is difficult. In some of these patients immunopathological reactions, induced by previous infections were probably the cause of the release of leucocytes. The leucocytes in semen were generally polymorphonuclear cells with altered membranes and in a few cases lymphocytes. Only sporadically agglomerations of leucocytes were found, as frequently observed in EPS. In the semen of patients with chronic prostatitis macrophages were rarely detected. More frequently these cells are found in cases of prostato-epididymitis.

More than 1000 colony forming units (CFU) of *Ureaplasma urealyticum* per ml of semen were detected in 8.6% of the patients. In 10% of the patients with markedly increased leucocyte counts (>5 million/ml of semen) the microbiological analysis revealed *N. gonorrhoeae,* the patients being asymptomatic at the time of investigation.

While a general agreement exists regarding the biochemical changes in semen of patients with chronic prostatitis, there is a considerable disagreement, concerning the influence of this disease on spermatogenesis. Statistical evaluations failed to reveal significant alterations of spermatozoa-counts, motility and morphology in the semen of fertility patients. But some patients showed pathological findings in semen analysis, which could be related to the chronic genital infection. This was concluded from improvement of spermatological findings after treatment of the infection and their impairment during relapses or reinfections.

The following phenomena were observed:

1. isolated *teratozoospermia* (amorphous heads, condensed heads) without impairment of spermatozoa-count and motility (STOLLA et al., 1978);
2. *exfoliative disorder of spermatogenesis* with increased numbers of spermatids in semen and a reduction of spermatozoa-count and alterations of their morphology. The morphological aberrations were characterized by a symmetric elongation of the postacrosomal segment of the spermatozoa-head, in more severe cases combined with deformations of this area, duplicate spermatozoa and defects of middlepeaces and tails (GOSLAR et al., 1982);
3. in advanced cases a heterogeneous testicular damage as *"mixed atrophy"*.

The spermatological findings of a patient with "non-specific" chronic prostatitis are shown in Table 1:

Table 1.

	Spermatozoa			Spermatids	Leucocytes
	count (Mio/ml)	motility (%)	morphology (%)	(%spermatozoa)	(Mio/ml)
1. NSGI*	103	55−60	43	22	1.1
2. Control after therapy	77.6	60	60	15	0.6
3. NSGI	56.0	60	35	31	1.0
4. Control after therapy	116.0	65−70	60	16	0.8

* non-specific genital infection (significant numbers of *U. urealyticum*).

A 25-year-old patient acquired two non-specific genital infections (urethro-prostatitis) during a period of 5 months. The first infection was externally treated with penicillin and subsequently with Trimethoprim-Sulfamethoxazol forte. Although there was a normal spermatozoa-count and motility, a marked increase in the number of exfoliated spermatids and a reduction in spermatozoa-morphology was present. The patient was treated with doxycycline 200 mg/daily for a period of two weeks. Two months later the spermatological findings were normal with the exception of a slight exfoliation of spermatids. After the second infection the exfoliative disorder was enhanced, the spermatozoa-morphology markedly altered. Again a normalization of the spermatological findings was achieved through therapy with doxycycline and anti-phlogistic drugs. The isomorphic impairment of the spermatological findings through the same disease reflecting an exfoliative disorder of spermatogenesis and the restoration through specific therapy indicate that the non-specific genital infection could have been the cause of the testicular disorder.

References

(1) GOSLAR, H. G., B. HILSCHER, S. G. HAIDER, N. HOFMANN, D. PASSIA, W. HILSCHER: Enzyme histochemical studies on the pathological changes in human Sertoli cells. J. Histochem. Cytochem. *30*: 1268−1274 (1982).
(2) HOFMANN, N.: Fertilitätsstörungen und chronische Entzündungen im Genitalbereich. In: SCHIRREN, C. (ed.): Fortschritte der Andrologie, Vol. 4. Grosse-Verlag, Berlin 1975.
(3) HOFMANN, N., L. WILSCH: Störungen der männlichen Fertilität bei unspezifischen chronischen Entzündungen der akzessorischen Genitaldrüsen. Therapiewoche *23*: 1998−2000 (1973).
(4) STOLLA, R., A. GROPP, W. LEIDL, N. HOFMANN: Teratozoospermie aus human- und tiermedizinischer Sicht. Hautarzt *29*: 518−524 (1978).

Abteilung für Geburtshilfe und Frauenheilkunde der Universität Kiel
und Michaelis-Hebammenschule
(Direktor: o. Prof. Dr. med. Dr. vet. h. c. K. Semm)

Leucocytospermia — A Sign for Chronic Infections of the Male Genital Tract?

H.-H. RIEDEL

During the evaluation of human semen using routine staining procedures, it is usually not very difficult to distinguish leucocytes from the cells of spermiogenesis. There is some disagreement concerning the frequency and significance of leucocytes in human semen (HEINKE and DOEPFMER, 1960; JOÈL, 1971). Little is known about the maximum number of leucocytes which can be present in the ejaculates of fertile men.

Difficulties in distinguishing leucocytes from polynuclear spermatides have led to the development of selective staining procedures for leucocytes: "Napth-

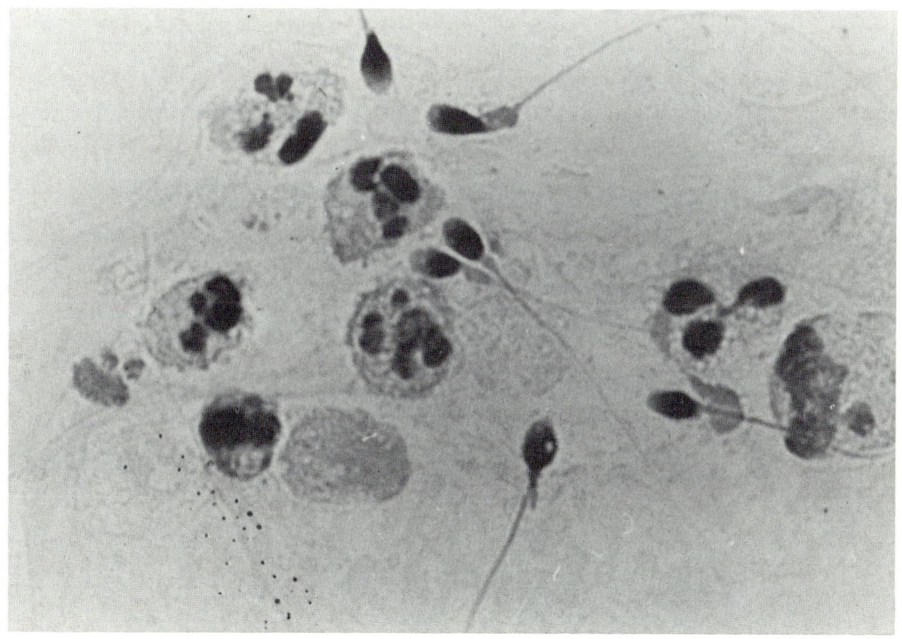

Fig. 1. Leucocytospermia (magnification 1200 times).

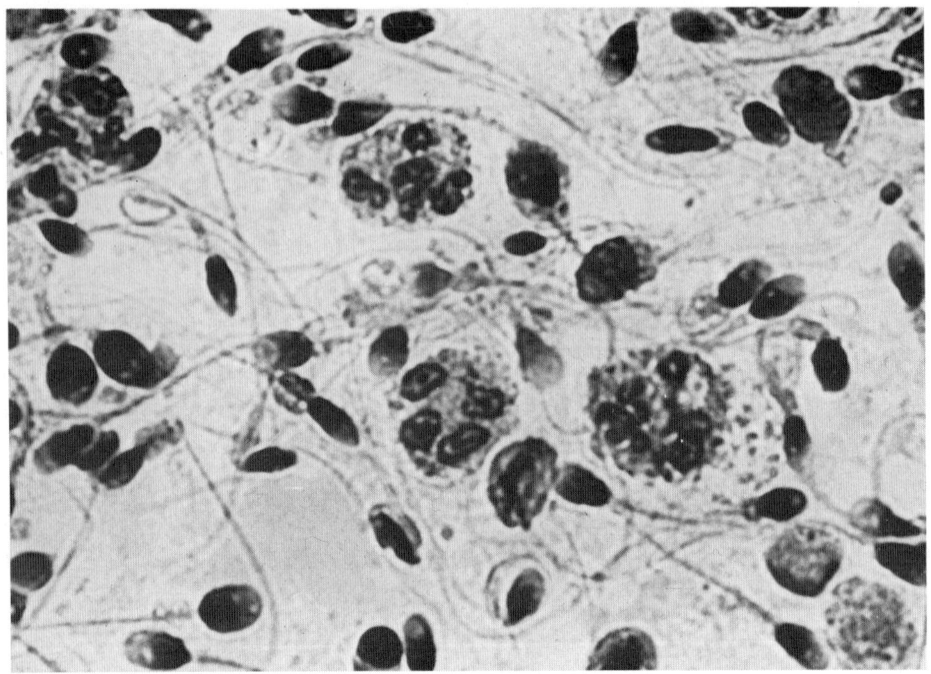

Fig. 2. Granulocytes and sperms by using Testsimplets (magnification 1200 times).

ol-Aminosäure-D-Chloracetat-technique" (ARONIS-BONN, 1964), "Benzidin-Cyanosin-technique" (ENDTZ, 1974), combination of Byran's sperm staining and Leishman's blood staining techniques (COUTURE et al., 1976) neutral-red-supravital-staining (PHADKE, 1978) (Fig. 1 and 2).

For the differentiation of round cells we used prestained microscope slides (Testsimplets) and the Cytur-Test strips, which also functioned as a rapid screening test for the detection of leucocytospermia. When leucocytospermia was detected, further cytological, bacteriological and immunological investigations were carried out in order to determine the cause. It is absolutely necessary to differentiate between patients with inflammatory disorders of the genitourinary tract as detected by other diagnostic measures, for example cases of chronic prostatitis, epididymitis etc., and patients who showed only a leucocytospermia. If there is any correlation with proven infections of the male genital tract such as prostatitis, epididymitis or spermatocystitis and the detection of leucocytes in the smear we speak about a so-called "pyospermia".

Using Testsimplets we were able to identify the leucocytes in all cases and to differentiate them from the spermiogenetic cells. The results obtained in the cytological differentiation of the ejaculates using Testsimplets were subsequently confirmed by routine Papanicolaou staining. Upon cytological evaluation of a group of 60 preparations with the diagnosis "normozoospermia" it was possible to demonstrate a leucocytospermia rate of 15% with the aid of Test-simplets. Subsequent assessment of the smears prepared by the Papanicolaou staining procedure confirmed the diagnosis of leucocytospermia in all cases.

Leucocytospermia is considered to exist if more than 2 million leucocytes per milliliter are detectable in the ejaculate or if, during microscopic differentiation at 400 × magnification, more than 3−5 leucocytes are detectable in each high power field. Leucocytospermia rates determined ejaculates from various diagnosis groups range from 10.5% to 15%. In seven cases of clear leucocytospermia we were able to confirm this finding using the Cytur-Test, i. e. there was a distinctive blue coloration of the previously white test area (Fig. 3 and 4).

From experience so far, however, it would appear that evaluated numbers of spermatogenetic cells or other round cells do not lead to a positive reaction of the test strips and thus cannot produce false-positive results. Granulocytes, which are the most commonly found type of leucocyte are easily differentiated from spermatogenetic cells with the use of Testsimplets. The special structures of the nucleus and cytoplasm of granulocytes clearly distinguishes them from the more round to oval spermatogenetic cells.

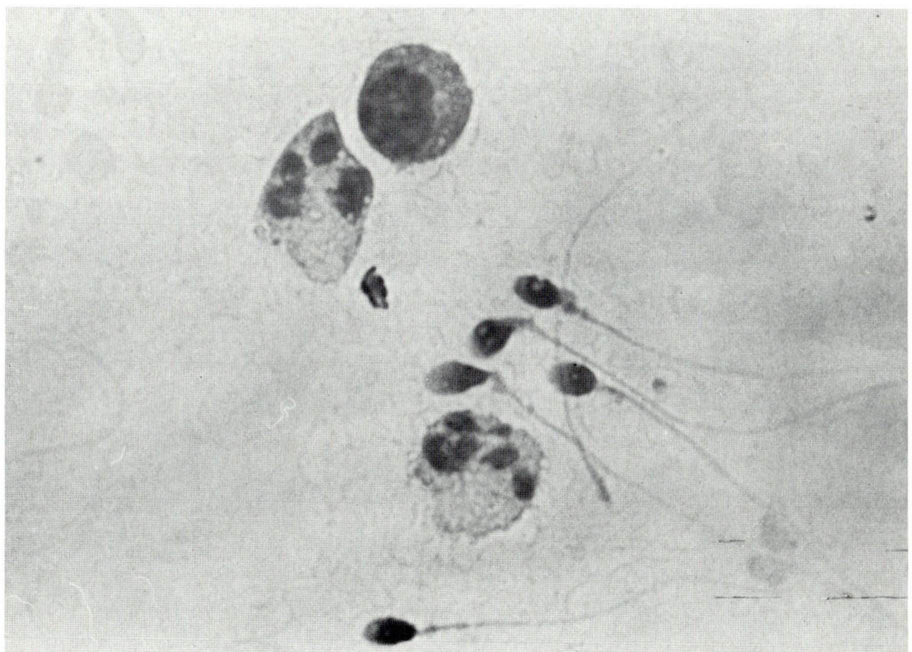

Fig. 3. Granulocytes and 1 spermatogonia. (Papanicolaon-colouring; magnification 1200 times.)

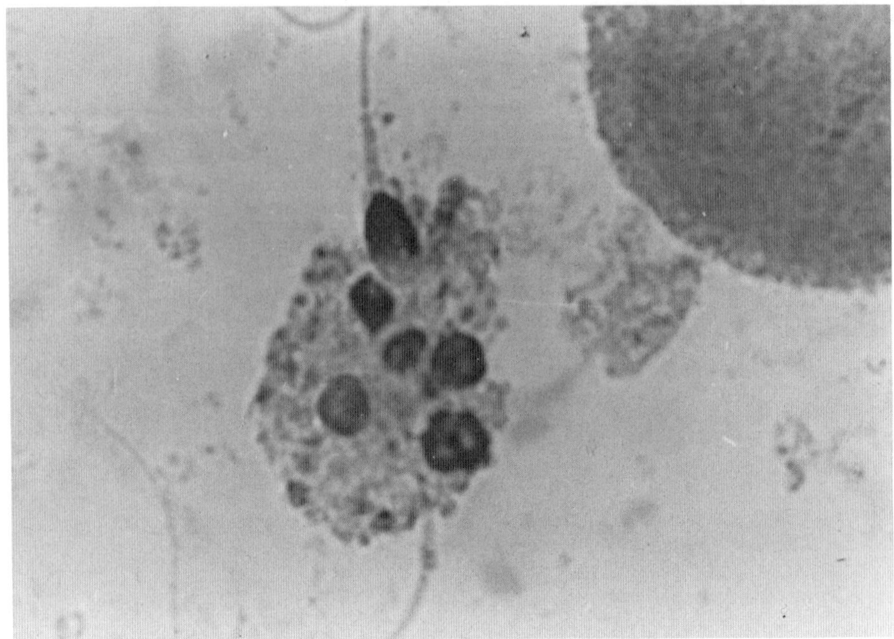

Fig. 4. Granulocyte with one phagocytosed spermhead. In the right upper corner a part of a spermatocyte. (Colouring by using Testsimplets; magnification 1600 times.)

As early as 1980, PURDY et al. and EDWARDS et al. required that the genital tract of a woman must be free of microorganisms, especially of "T-Mycoplasmas" before admission to the in vitro fertilization program and that examination of the husband's ejaculate must prove the absence of pathogenic microorganisms. Antibiotic treatment is therefore recommended if these requirements are not fulfilled, by these authors, as well as, by JONES, 1981; FEICHTINGER, 1981; TROUNSON, 1981 and other groups.

In 1979 NIKKANEN et al. published that "the most common finding in the semen of the group of patients with semen infections, was a slight or moderate oligo-astheno-teratozoospermia. The sperm count, the percentage of spermatozoa with normal morphology was significantly lower in the group exhibiting a dormant infection. The presence of leucocytosis among infected semen was obvious." The authors found a temporary reduction in the number of leucocytes after treatment with tetracyclines but also a partially negative effect on the motility of spermatozoa.

HOFMAN et al. reported in 1981 that 20% of infertile patients had increased number of leucocytes in the semen without expressing symptoms of a chronic prostatitis or other genital infections. Similar results were found by RIEDEL and

Schirren, 1978. We observed in about 10–15% of ejaculates from patients of the sterility consultation hours a so-called "leucocytospermia" which did not clearly correlate with the results of the bacteriological examination of the semen.

In 1977 Frazer and Taylor-Robinson infected mouse oocytes and spermatozoa artificially with mycoplasmas. A statistically significant reduction of in vitro fertilization rates was obtained associated with a significant "reduction in embryonic development in the treated groups when compared with the untreated group".

Using the hamster oocyte human sperm system, we were able to show in 1981 a correlation between the occurrence of pathogenic bacteria in ejaculates and a decrease of penetration rates, as well as, degeneration of hamster ova. With 5 ejaculates of the category normozoospermia which were found to contain bacterial numbers greater than 10^5/ml, which were identified to be staphylococci (1 ×), enterococci (1 ×), *Escherichia coli* (1 ×) and mycoplasmas (2 ×), no penetration of inseminated zona pellucida free hamster oocytes occurred.

Another remarkable observation within this system was the fact that ejaculates with high concentrations of leucocytes produced significantly lower penetration rates when compared to ejaculates with few or no leucocytes. Average penetration rates dropped clearly with leucocyte concentrations of more than 3% in the original ejaculate; leucocyte concentrations of more than 10% resulted in a penetration rate of 0% whereas leucocyte concentrations of less than 0.5% produced average penetration rates of 36%. Since the leucocytes within the seminal plasma were removed through the different washing steps routinely carried out for insemination of zona free hamster ova, the presence of certain microorganisms probably anaerobic species should be considered which could be sticking to the spermatozoa surface thus causing the described changes and may therefore account for the decrease of penetration rates. Up to now electronmicroscopic studies for clarification of this matter are not available.

The clear correlation between positive bacteriological findings or the massive occurrence of leucocytes in ejaculates used for insemination and decreased penetration rates seen in the hamster oocyte human sperm system were not demonstrated during fertilization of human oocytes.

In 1982 we started a systematic bacteriological examination of ejaculates to be used for in vitro fertilization: A total of 166 ejaculates from patients taking part in the in vitro fertilization program were examined. In 70 ejaculates (42%) bacteria numbers greater than 10^5/ml were found. 96 (58%) of the probes were negative or had bacteria numbers less than 10^4/ml. Mycoplasmas were found in 37 of the examined ejaculates or 22.3%. The second most frequent group of microorganisms were enterococci found in 17 patients (10.2%).

When considering sperm quality and positive, as well as negative bacteriological findings with regards to the fertilization rate of human oocytes the following results were obtained: After insemination of one or more pelviscopically obtained oocytes with sperm of the husband in 16 out of 24 cases, with bacteria numbers greater than 10^5/ml, the cleavage of at least one oocyte occurred leading to an embryo transfer rate of 66.7%. Of these 16 cases in which microbiological examinations were positive, cleavage and embryo transfer of inseminated oocytes took place even though 10 cases (62.5%) were observed in which all inseminated oocytes were fertilized. 10 of the 16 ejaculates with positive bacteria culture but fertilizing inseminated oocytes belonged to the normozoospermic category (62.5%), only 1 showed a high grade oligozoospermia. Of the 8 ejaculates of the group not effecting fertilization 6 (75%) were pathologic and only two belonged to the normozoospermic category. 19 of 37 ejaculates with negative bacteriological finding (51.4%) fertilized at least one of the inseminated oocytes, 11 of these 19 ejaculates (57.9%) belonged to the normozoospermic category, while the other showed a more or less clear pathospermia.

Of the 19 bacteriologically negative ejaculates not fertilizing the obtained oocytes only 7 (38.9%) belonged to the normozoospermic category, while 12 were clearly pathologic. 11 of the 19 ejaculates of this group fertilizing at least one of the pelviscopically obtained oocytes succeeded in fertilizing all obtained oocytes (57.1%).

From results obtained to date any direct effect of microbial contamination on sperm in the human in vitro fertilization system cannot be demonstrated. The cleavage and embryo transfer rates within the group having positive bacteriological findings in the sperm were even higher than within the group with negative bacteriological findings. But the 13 pregnancies we have obtained all resulted from bacteria free sperm. When discussing the extracorporal fertilization of human oocytes it is not certain if contaminated sperm may effect degeneration of embryos at a later stage thus resulting in no pregnancies, taking into consideration results obtained by FRAZER and TAYLOR-ROBINSON in the animal experiment. According to the results published by FISHEL in 1981, a reduction of implantation rates after application of bacteria contaminated ejaculates for insemination can also not be excluded.

In our study no statistically significant correlation between positive or negative bacteriological findings and the andrological category and cytology of the ejaculate smears were found. Remarkably, no correlation existed between the so-called "leucocytospermia" and positive bacteriological findings.

Groups of bacteria not always detectable during routine andrological diagnosis − as for example certain species of anaerobic organisms − may be perhaps responsible for the occurrence of leucocytospermia.

No correlation existed between special groups of bacteria, andrological diagnosis and differential spermiocytogramms. The most common germs detected by microbiological examinations such as "T-mycoplasmas" and enterococci, were found in ejaculates of the normozoospermic category, as well as, in pathological ejaculates and these were not associated with specific cytological changes. We are therefore unable to confirm the correlation reported by Derrick and Dahlberg, 1976 between increasing leucocyte concentrations and decreasing sperm quality, which was used to explain the inter-relation between infections of male genital tract and reduced fertility rates.

The existence of leucocytes or of leucocytospermia within the ejaculate is not correlated with special inflammations of the male genital tract. Likewise a statistically justified relationship between reduced fertilization and the occurrence of certain species of bacteria within the ejaculate was not found. Even in leucocyte-free ejaculates numbers of microorganisms greater than 10^5/ml were demonstrated and leucocytospermia was detectable with negative bacteriological findings.

The evaluation of smears of normozoospermic men showed a clear leucocytospermia in 15% of patients, without having any correlation to sperm bacteriology. These patients have to be differentiated from patients where the detection of leucocytes in the semen smear is correlated with a proven prostatitis, epididymitis etc. In these cases we speak about a pyospermia.

It can be said that there is no relation between microbiological and cytological findings of ejaculates used for insemination of oocytes and the obtained fertilization, cleavage and embryo transfer rates in the human in vitro fertilization program here. But since a negative effect on implantation rates or embryonic development cannot be excluded, detailed bacteriological examinations and probably antibiotic treatment may be recommended before admission into an in vitro fertilization program.

References

(1) Aronis-Bonn, E.: Beitrag zur Cytodiagnostik der Leukozyten im Ejakulat beim primären Hodenschaden. Klin. exp. Derm. *219*: 935−937 (1964).

(2) Couture, M., M. Ulstein, J. Leonhard, C. H. Paulsen: Improved staining method for differentiation immature germ cells from white blond cells in human seminal fluid. Andrologia *8*: 61−66 (1976).

(3) Derrick, F. C., B. Dahlberg: Male genital tract infections and sperm viability. In: Hafez, E. S. E.: Human semen and fertility regulation in men. Mosby, Saint Louis 1976.

(4) Edwards, R. G., P. C. Steptoe, J. M. Purdy: Establishing full-term human pregnancies using cleaving embryos grown in vitro. Brit. J. Obstet. Gynaec. *87*: 737−756 (1980).

(5) Endtz, A. W.: A rapid staining method for differentiating granulocytes from "Germinal cells" in Papanicolaou-stained semen. Acta Cytol. *18*: 2−7 (1974).

(6) FEICHTINGER, W., S. SZALAY, P. KEMETER, A. BECK, H. JANISCH: In vitro Fertilisierung menschlicher Eizellen sowie Embryotransfer. Geburtsh. Frauenheilkd. *41*: 482−489 (1981).

(7) FISHEL, S. B., R. G. EDWARDS: Essential of fertilization. In: EDWARDS R. G., J. M. PURDY: Human conception in vitro; pp. 157−174. 1982.

(8) FRAZER, L. R., D. TAYLOR-ROBINSON: The effect of mycoplasma pulmonis on fertilization and preimplantation development in vitro of mouse eggs. Fertil. Steril. *28*: 488−498 (1977).

(9) HEINKE, E., R. DOEPFMER: Fertilitätsstörungen beim Manne. Somatischer Teil. In: JADERSSOHN, J.: Handbuch der Haut- und Geschlechtskrankheiten. Erg. Werk Bd. VI/3. Springer, Berlin−Göttingen−Heidelberg 1960.

(10) HOFMANN, N.: Fertilitätsstörungen und chronische Entzündungen im Genitalbereich. Fortschritte der Andrologie, Vol. 4. Grosse Verlag, Berlin 1975.

(11) JOEL, C. A.: The etiology of male fertility disturbances. In: JOEL, C. A.: Fertility disturbances in men and women; pp. 71−74. Karger, Basel 1971.

(12) JONES, H.: Discussion on the fertilization of human oocytes in vivo and in vitro. In: EDWARDS, R. G., J. M. PURDY: Human conception in vitro; pp. 191−200. 1982.

(13) NIKKANEN, V., M. GRÖNROOS, J. SUOMINEN, S. MULTAMÄKI: Silent infection in male accessory genital organs and male infertility. Andrologia *11*: 236−241 (1979).

(14) PHADKE, A. M.: Neutral red supravital staining for cellular elements in the semen. Andrologia *10*: 80−84 (1978).

(15) PURDY, J. M.: Pregnancies with embryos grown in vitro. Brit. J. Obstet. Gynaec. *87*: 757−768 (1980).

(16) PURDY, J. M.: Methods for fertilization and embryo culture in vitro. In: EDWARDS R. G., J. M. PURDY: Human conception in vitro; pp. 135−156. 1982.

(17) RIEDEL, H.-H., C. SCHIRREN: Untersuchungen zur Differenzierung der Rundzellen im menschlichen Ejakulat. Z. Hautkr. *53*: 255−267 (1978).

(18) RIEDEL, H.-H.: Techniques for the detection of leucocytospermia in human semen. Arch. of Androl. *5*: 287−293 (1980).

(19) RIEDEL, H.-H., K. SEMM: Über den Nachweis der Leukozytospermie und deren Bedeutung für die Fertilität des Mannes. Z. Hautkr. *55*: 897−1006 (1980).

(20) RIEDEL, H.-H.: Grenzanforderungen an Ejakulate, die für die extra-corporale Befruchtung verwendet werden sollen. Zuchthygiene *3*: 101 (1982).

(21) RIEDEL, H.-H., V. BAUKLOH, L. METTLER: Die Bedeutung der Sperma-Qualität für die in vitro Fertilisation − Ergebnisse von Untersuchungen im Humansystem und im zona pellucida freien Hamstereizellsystem. Andrologia *15:* 595−604 (1983).

(22) TROUNSON, A. O., C. A. SHIVERS, R. McMASTERS, A LOPATA: Inhibition of spermbinding and fertilization of human ova by antibodies to porcine zona pellucida and by human sera. Arch. of Antrol. *4*: 29−36 (1980).

(23) TROUNSON, A.O.: Factors influencing the success of fertilization and embryonic growth in vitro. In: EDWARDS, R. G., J. M. PURDY: Human conception in vitro; pp. 201−207. 1982.

Urologische Klinik, Abteilung Andrologie, Institut für Medizinische Mikrobiologie,
Klinikum der Justus-Liebig-Universität Gießen

Semen Quality in Men with Urogenital Infections by Ureaplasma urealyticum

W. WEIDNER, W. KRAUSE, H. BRUNNER, H. G. SCHIEFER

Introduction

Genitourinary tract infections are regarded as major pathogenetic factors for male infertility. The two most important mechanisms are assumed to be: 1. direct effect on sperm function by the microorganisms, 2. secretory dysfunction of the male sexual glands after infection (CALDAMONE and COCKETT, 1978). Whereas bacterial infections of the male genitourinary tract by gram-negative bacteria, e. g. *E.coli,* have been investigated extensively, the role of mycoplasmas in diseases of male reproductive organs is debatable until now. This insufficient understanding is due to the unestablished role of these microorganisms in prostatitis, which is still a subject of urological research (FRIBERG, 1979).

Review of literature

Four different species of mycoplasmas are known to colonize the male urogenital tract: *Ureaplasma (U.) urealyticum, Mycoplasma (M.) hominis, Mycoplasma (M.) fermentans* and *Mycoplasma (M.) genitalium* (TAYLOR-ROBINSON and McCORMACK, 1980). At present only *U. urealyticum* can be considered a facultative pathogen in male lower urinary tract infections (BRUNNER et al., 1983). For another recently detected mycoplasma species, *Mycoplasma genitalium,* a similar role has not yet been established (TAYLOR-ROBINSON et al., 1981).

Because mycoplasmas can be detected in the anterior urethra of up to 50 percent of healthy men (TAYLOR-ROBINSON and McCORMACK, 1980), mere isolation of these microorganisms from urogenital tract secretions does not permit to draw any conclusion on their etiologic role in a special disease unless a pure culture of mycoplasmas is obtained from normally sterile tissue. Using a quantitative cultivation technique for ureaplasmas (BRUNNER et al., 1983) we were

Table 1. Characteristic distribution pattern of ureaplasmas in urethral discharge, urine specimens, and EPS in healthy men and in men with urethritis or prostatitis.

	Urethral discharge	VB1	VB2	EPS	VB3
	cfu/ml	cfu/ml	cfu/ml	cfu/ml	cfu/ml
Healthy controls	−	$<10^3$	$<10^3$	$<10^4$	$<10^3$
Urethritis	$\geq 10^4$	$\geq 10^3$	−	−	−
Prostatitis	−	$<10^3$	$<10^3$	$\geq 10^4$	$\geq 10^3$

VB1 = first voided urine, VB2 = mid-stream urine, EPS = prostatic secretions, VB3 = urine after prostatic massage.

able to demonstrate significantly high ureaplasma numbers in urethral discharge and first voided urine in patients with nongonococcal urethritis (WEIDNER et al., 1978, 1982) and in prostatic secretions and urine voided after prostatic massage of patients with "non-bacterial" prostatitis (WEIDNER et al., 1978; 1980; BRUNNER et al., 1983), when compared with healthy controls (WEIDNER et al., 1982; BRUNNER et al., 1983) (Table 1).

Whereas in healthy men numbers of ureaplasmas were always $<10^3$ colony forming units (cfu) per ml of first voided urine (VB1), the organisms were detected in men with urethritis and "non-bacterial" prostatitis in a characteristic distribution-pattern (Table 1). In these cases only, tetracycline therapy proved to be effective by disappearance of symptoms and eradication of the microorganisms (WEIDNER et al., 1978; BRUNNER et al., 1983), whereas in cases with lower numbers, ureaplasmas must be considered commensals of the anterior urethra.

In our opinion, this quantitative analysis is at present the most practicable diagnostic technique to provide evidence for the etiologic role of ureaplasmas in urogenital tract diseases. The mere isolation of ureaplasmas from semen specimens may be misleading, because the specimens might have been contaminated during passage of the ejaculate through the urethra colonized by ureaplasmas (HARGREAVE et al., 1982). These difficulties should be kept in mind in the controversial discussion about the role of ureaplasmas in male fertility.

Ureaplasmas have been discussed to be involved in male infertility, since early microscopic observations had demonstrated that these microorganisms attach to spermatozoa (GNARPE and FRIBERG, 1973). According to these findings decreased sperm motility had been postulated as evidence for the presence of ureaplasmas in semen specimens (FOLWKES et al., 1975). Additionally, the authors described increasing alterations of motility, sperm density, and morphology in semen samples infected by ureaplasmas as compared with ureaplasma-free specimens (FOLWKES et al., 1975; O'LEARY and FRICK, 1975; SWENSON et al., 1979; TOTH et al., 1978). Furthermore, tetracycline therapy of patients with ureaplasma infected semen samples appeared to improve semen quality, especially the motility of sperms (SWENSON et al., 1979). However, all these data have not been confirmed by others (DESAI et al., 1980; CINTRON et al., 1981; TAYLOR-ROBINSON et al., 1983).

Considering this controversial discussion a study of ejaculate parameters in well-established cases of prostatitis caused by *Ureaplasma urealyticum* in comparison with men suffering from prostatodynia was started in order to further investigate the role of these microorganisms in ejaculate quality and male fertility.

Patients, methods

From 1975–1980 a standardized diagnostic procedure was performed in 597 men, suffering from prostatitis (BRUNNER und WEIDNER, 1983). In addition to quantitative mycoplasma determination following the "four-specimen-technique" (MEARES and STAMEY, 1968), 412 ejaculate samples of these patients were analyzed for common bacteria and mycoplasmas. In 127 cases the microbiological analysis was possible as a direct follow-up study, i.e., ejaculate analysis and "four-specimen-technique" were performed during a 6 hour period.

Semen analysis: Cultivation and identification of microorganisms were as detailed previously (WEIDNER et al., 1978, 1982; BRUNNER et al., 1983). Prolonged incubation as required for isolation of *M. genitalium* was not performed. The routinely done sperm analysis included the following parameters: sperm count, motility, morphology, fructose concentration, numbers of "round cells" (i.e. all leucocytes and spermatides) and erythrocytes (KRAUSE and ROTHAUGE, 1981). Determination of zinc was performed by atomic absorption spectrophotometry. The entire seminal fluid, including spermatozoa, was used for the analysis (STURM, 1981).

Classification of prostatitis: Prostatitis was defined by the presence of common bacteria (gramnegative rods, enterococci) and *Ureaplasma urealyticum* in the following numbers: VB1 and VB2 $<10^3$ cfu/ml; EPS $\geq 10^4$ cfu/ml; VB3 $\geq 10^3$ cfu/ml (Table 1). Prostatic inflammatory response was diagnosed by counting leucocytes in EPS and granulocytes in VB3. In EPS ≥ 10 leucocytes per microscopic field at 1000-fold magnification, and in VB3 ≥ 4 granulocytes per microscopic field at 400-fold magnification were considered pathognomonic for prostatitis (WEIDNER and EBNER, 1984). Only patients with ureaplasma-associated prostatitis were considered for fertility analysis; men suffering from common bacterial infection and with evidence of *Chlamydia trachomatis* were excluded. Prostatodynia was defined by the absence of significant numbers of bacteria and leucocytes.

Results

Microbiologic findings in ejaculate specimens (Table 2): In the 412 ejaculate specimens analyzed for mycoplasmas, *U. urealyticum* was the most frequently detected species. In 46 cases (11.2%) the number of cfu/ml was $>10^3$, none of these patients had a monoinfection by *M. hominis*.

Ureaplasma determinations in ejaculate and "four-specimen-technique" (Table 3): In 27 men with ureaplasma-associated prostatitis (for classification, see Table 1) a microbiologic analysis of the ejaculate specimens could be performed at the same time. *U. urealyticum* was detected in all ejaculate samples. But in 10 of these 27 men, numbers of ureaplasmas did not exceed the lower limit of 10^3 cfu/ml ejaculate, which we consider normal contamination from urethral colonization. In contrast, in prostatodynia ureaplasma numbers in ejaculate did not differ from cultural findings in healthy controls.

Table 2. Isolation rates and quantitative determination of ureaplasmas in 412 ejaculate specimens.

No. of organisms isolated (cfu/ml)	U.urealyticum or M.hominis	U.urealyticum (monoinfection)	U.urealyticum + M.hominis	M.hominis (monoinfection)	no mycoplasmas detected
Total	128 (31%)	104 (25.2%)	15 (3.6%)	9 (2.2%)	284 (69%)
$<10^3$	28	71	2	9	
10^3-10^4	30	23	7	–	
$>10^4$	16	10	6	–	

Table 3. Numbers of *U. urealyticum* in ejaculate specimens of patients with urogenital diseases classified by using the "four-specimen-technique", and healthy controls.

Ureaplasma numbers in ejaculate (cfu/ml)	Ureaplasma-associated prostatitis (n = 27)	Prostatodynia (n = 25)	Healthy men (n = 23)
$<10^3$	10	8	9
10^3-10^4	5	–	–
$>10^4$	12	–	–

Table 4. Correlation between numbers of ureaplasmas in ejaculate samples and common ejaculate parameters.

	Number of specimens analyzed	r	t
Volume (ml)	342	−0.055	1.02
Sperm density (mill/ml)	403	−0.009	0.18
Motility (%)	384	0.052	1.04
Abnormal morphology (%)	359	−0.060	1.15
Round cells (mill/ml)	349	−0.016	0.30
Erythrocytes (mill/ml)	372	−0.036	0.70
Fructose (μmol/ml)	342	−0.104	1.93
Zinc (μg/ml)	160	−0.510	3.41*

* zinc: negative significant correlation; r = 0.510; t-test gives p ≤ 0.01 (r = correlation coefficient; t = T-value).

Quantitative determination of U. urealyticum and ejaculate parameters (Table 4): The comparison between the numbers of ureaplasmas and the results of ejaculate analysis did not reveal a statistically significant correlation with volume, sperm density, motility, abnormal morphology, number of round cells and erythrocytes. In contrast a significantly negative correlation between the numbers of ureaplasmas and zinc concentration in seminal fluid and an almost identical, but not significant correlation to the content of fructose were found.

Cellular and humoral ejaculate parameters and ureaplasma associated prostatitis (Table 5): The number of round cells was the only cellular parameter which showed a significant difference as compared with prostatodynia. The evaluation of numbers of round cells exhibited a significant increase in ureaplasma-associated prostatitis. Both parameters of secretory dysfunction, i.e. fructose content and zinc level, were decreased significantly.

Table 5. Median values, 25 and 75 percentile values (in parenthesis), in ureaplasma-associated prostatitis and prostatodynia.

	n	Ureaplasma-associated prostatitis	n	Prostatodynia
Volume (ml)	71	4 (2.0−5.0)	41	4 (3.0−5.0)
Sperm density (mill/ml)	96	50 (24.5−88)	63	49 (18−86)
Motility (%)	58	58 (45−70)	59	57 (35−68)
Abnormal morphology (%)	86	26 (19−35)	47	29 (22−36)
Round cells (mill/ml)	91	0.9* (0.4−1.5)	49	0.4 (0.0−1.2)
Erythrocytes (mill/ml)	92	0 (0−0.5)	51	0 (0.0−0.0)
Fructose (μmol/ml)	78	12* (8−16)	46	14.5 (9−21)
Zinc (μg/ml)	23	115* (18−318)	79	166 (51−928)

* significant difference (u-Test) between ureaplasma-associated prostatitis and prostatodynia (p ≤ 0.05).

Discussion

The most important problem in microbiologic studies of male infertility remains "to distinguish the mere presence of ureaplasmas in semen samples as result of contamination during passage through the urethra at the time of ejaculation from their etiologic role in infertility" (HARGREAVE et al., 1982).

This question can only be answered by performing isolation studies and relating their results to semen parameters. Ureaplasma numbers of $< 10^3$ cfu/ml of ejaculate are regarded to correspond to the contamination from urethral colonization of normal men. In the present study only in 11.2% of all ejaculate specimens, the number of ureaplasmas exceeded 10^3 cfu per ml of sample. Accordingly, in prostatodynia numbers of ureaplasmas in ejaculate were always $< 10^3$ per ml. Semen specimens in cases of ureaplasma-associated prostatitis classified by the "four-specimen-technique", did not reveal higher numbers of *U. urealyticum* in all cases. This fact may depend upon the varying portion of male genital gland secretions in ejaculate (DAHLBERG, 1976) and is well known from common bacterial prostatitis (MOBLEY, 1975). Although numbers of ureaplasmas were not always greater than the critical value of $> 10^3$, the number of round cells as parameter of inflammatory reaction in ejaculate was significantly increased in all cases of ureaplasma-associated prostatitis. This leucocytal reaction had been demonstrated similarly in prostatic secretions (WEIDNER and EBNER, 1984).

To the best of our knowledge, other studies concerning secretory dysfunction of the accessory glands in ureaplasmal infections have not been published. Both parameters of secretory dysfunction, i.e. fructose content and zinc levels were significantly decreased. These findings correspond to the well-accepted hypothesis of disturbed secretory capacity of the accessory genital glands in common bacterial prostatitis (ELIASSON, 1968; COLLEEN et al., 1975). As in disease caused by common bacteria, two explanations may be discussed: 1. chronic inflammation already exists and is followed by increased multiplication of ureaplasmas, since zinc with its antibacterial activity is diminished by the preceding inflammation (FAIR et al., 1976), or 2. ureaplasmas infect the gland and cause inflammatory reactions with decreased zinc and fructose levels in fluids of prostatic gland and seminal vesicles (MEARES, 1983).

Similar to other studies with (HOFMANN et al., 1979; TAYLOR-ROBINSON et al., 1983) or without quantitative ureaplasma determination (DESAI et al., 1980; CINTRON et al., 1981) in men with ureaplasmal infections of the urogenital tract, we found that volume, sperm density, motility, and range of abnormal morphology *did not differ* from values in prostatodynia. Additionally our data correspond to those of a clinical investigation, that, in patients with proven male infertility, high numbers of ureaplasmas are very rarely detected in semen samples ($\sim 8.6\%$) (HOFMANN et al., 1983). However, recent investigations in women, characterized by "infertility with a male factor", have demonstrated a prevalence of ureaplasmal infections as compared with other infertile populations (CASSELL et al., 1983). In our opinion these data stress the necessity of further studies on the role of these microorganisms under the special aspect of male-female interactions.

Acknowledgement

The skillful assistance of Mrs. S. PETERS is gratefully acknowledged.

References

(1) BRUNNER, H., W. WEIDNER, H. G. SCHIEFER: Studies on the role of Ureaplasma urealyticum and Mycoplasma hominis in prostatitis. J. Inf. Dis. *147*: 807 (1983).

(2) BRUNNER, H., W. WEIDNER: Ureaplasma urealyticum und chronische Prostatitis. In: BRUNNER, H., W. KRAUSE, C. F. ROTHAUGE, W. WEIDNER (eds.): Chronische Prostatitis; pp. 69—76. Schattauer, Stuttgart—New York 1983.

(3) CALDAMONE, A. A., A. T. K. COCKETT: Infertility and genitourinary infection. Urology *12*: 304 (1978).

(4) CASSELL, G. H., J. B. YOUNGER, M. B. BROWN, R. E. BLACKWELL, J. R. DAVIS, P. MARRIOTT, S. STAGNO: Microbiologic studies in infertile women at the time of diagnostic laparoscopy. New Engl. J. Med. *308*: 502 (1983).

(5) CINTRON, R. D., J. W. E. WORTHAM, A. ACOSTA: The association of semen factors with the recovery of Ureaplasma urealyticum. Fert. Steril *36*: 648 (1981).

(6) COLLEEN, S., P. A. MÂRDH, S. SCHYTZ: Magnesium and Zinc in seminal fluid of healthy males and patients with non-acute prostatitis with and without gonorrhoeae. Scand. J. Urol. Nephrol. *9*: 192 (1975).

(7) DAHLBERG, B.: Asymptomatic bacteriospermia. Urology *13*: 563 (1976).

(8) DESAI, SH., M. C. COHEN, M. KHATAMEE, E. LEITER: Ureaplasma urealyticum infection: does it have a role in male infertility? J. Urol. *124*: 469 (1980).

(9) ELIASSON, R.: Biochemical analysis of human semen in the study of the physiology and pathophysiology of the male accessory genital glands. Fert. Steril. *19*: 344 (1968).

(10) FAIR, W. R., J. COUCH, N. WEHNER: Prostatic antibacterial factor. Urology *12*: 169 (1976).

(11) FOLWKES, D. M., G. B. DOOHER, W. M. O'LEARY: Evidence by scanning electron microscopy for an association between spermatozoa and T-mycoplasmas in men of infertile marriage. Fertil. Steril. *26*: 1203 (1975).

(12) FRIBERG, J.: Mycoplasmas and infertility. Curr. Ther. Res. *26*: 760 (1979).

(13) GNARPE, H., J. FRIBERG: T-mycoplasmas on spermatozoa and infertility. Nature (London) *254*: 97 (1973).

(14) HARGREAVE, T. B., M. TORRANCE, H. YOUNG, A. B. HARIS: Isolation of Ureaplasma urealyticum from seminal plasma in relation to sperm antibody levels and sperm motility. Andrologia *14*: 223 (1982).

(15) HOFMANN, N., H. BRUNNER, U. MEISEL: Zur Bedeutung von Ureaplasma urealyticum im Sperma von Fertilitätspatienten. Z. Hautkr. *54*: 147 (1979).

(16) HOFMANN, N., H. BRUNNER, G. HAMMER, O. KURZ: Klinische, spermatologische und mikrobiologische Befunde bei Fertilitätspatienten mit chronischer Prostatitis. In: BRUNNER, H., W. KRAUSE, C. F. ROTHAUGE, W. WEIDNER (eds.): Chronische Prostatitis; pp. 183−187. Schattauer, Stuttgart−New York 1983.

(17) KRAUSE, W., C. F. ROTHAUGE (eds.): Andrologische Erkrankungen der männlichen Geschlechtsorgane. Enke, Stuttgart 1981.

(18) O'LEARY, W. M., J. FRICK: The correlation of human male infertility with the presence of mycoplasma T-strains. Andrologia 7: 309 (1975).

(19) MEARES, E. M., T. A. STAMEY: Bacteriologic localization patterns in bacterial prostatitis and urethritis. Invest. Urol. 5: 492 (1968).

(20) MEARES, E. M.: Chronische bakterielle Prostatitis. In: H. BRUNNER, W. KRAUSE, C. F. ROTHAUGE, W. WEIDNER (eds.): Chronische Prostatitis; pp. 3−15. Schattauer, Stuttgart−New York 1983.

(21) MOBLEY, D. F.: Semen cultures in the diagnosis of bacterial prostatitis. J. Urol. 114: 83 (1975).

(22) SWENSON, CH. E., A. TOTH, W. M. O'LEARY: Ureaplasma urealyticum and human infertility: the effect of antibiotic therapy on semen quality. Fertil. Steril. 31: 660 (1979).

(23) STURM, J.: Zink im Ejakulat bei chronischer Prostatitis. Inauguraldissertation, Gießen 1980.

(24) TAYLOR-ROBINSON, D., W. C. MCCORMACK: The genital mycoplasmas. New Engl. J. Med. 302: 1063 (1980).

(25) TAYLOR-ROBINSON, D., J. G. TULLY, P. M. FURR, R. M. COLE, D. L. ROSE, D. F. HANNA: Urogenital mycoplasma infections of man: a review with observations on a recently discovered mycoplasma. Isr. J. Med. Sci. 17: 524 (1981).

(26) TAYLOR-ROBINSON, D., P. E. MUNDAY, N. F. HANNA, B. J. THOMAS, P. M. FURR: Mikrobiologische Aspekte der nicht-gonorrhoischen Urethroprostatitis und ihre wahrscheinlichen Konsequenzen. In: BRUNNER, H., W. KRAUSE, C. F. ROTHAUGE, W. WEIDNER (eds.): Chronische Prostatitis; pp. 53−60. Schattauer, Stuttgart−New York 1983.

(27) TOTH, A., C. E. SWENSON, W. M. O'LEARY: Light microscopy as an aid in predicting ureaplasma infection in human semen. Fertil. Steril. 30: 586 (1978).

(28) WEIDNER, W., H. BRUNNER, W. KRAUSE, C. F. ROTHAUGE: Zur Bedeutung von Ureaplasma urealyticum bei unspezifischer Prostato-Urethritis. Dtsch. med. Wschr. 103: 465 (1978).

(29) WEIDNER, W., H. BRUNNER, W. KRAUSE: Quantitative culture of Ureaplasma urealyticum in patients with chronic prostatitis or prostatosis. J. Urol. 124: 622 (1980).

(30) WEIDNER, W., H. G. SCHIEFER, H. KRAUSS, J. ENGSTFELD: Untersuchungen zur Ätiologie der nicht-gonorrhoischen Urethritis. Dtsch. med. Wschr. 107: 1227 (1982).

(31) WEIDNER, W., H. EBNER: Cytological analysis of urine after prostatic massage (VB3) − a new technique for a discrimination diagnosis of prostatitis. In: BRUNNER, H., W. KRAUSE, C. F. ROTHAUGE, W. WEIDNER (eds.): Chronic prostatitis; pp. 141−151. Schattauer, Stuttgart−New York 1984.

Gynaecological Endocrinology Unit, "La Carità" Hospital, Locarno
Andrology Unit, Urology Department, Microbiological Laboratory and Pathology Department
Provincial Hospital Magenta, Milan

Electrophoretical Analyses of Human Expressed Prostatic Secretion (EPS) and the Diagnosis of Prostatitis

M. BALERNA, G. M. COLPI, A. CAMPANA, L. ROVEDA, A. TOMMASINI-DEGNA, A. ZANOLLO

Introduction

Despite considerable efforts, our knowledge about the intimate interactions between seminal plasma components and spermatozoa at or after ejaculation is scanty. Many authors, however, agree today in postulating direct interactions between this complex fluid and the gamete cells [see e.g. (11, 13, 15) and references therein]. It can easily be predicted, in such a context, that any "anomaly" in the seminal plasma composition induced by pathologies of the internal genitalia should be analyzed in view of its potential effect(s) on spermatozoa (4, 6, 14). During high-resolution studies on seminal plasma proteins, we were struck by the many inter- and intra-individual proteinic pattern variabilities we could not explain without admitting an altered proteic contribution from the male accessory sex glands (1). We began therefore to study in some detail the high-resolution protein patterns of expressed prostatic secretion (EPS) obtained from urologic and infertile patients clinically suspected to have prostatic inflammation. The present report will focus on some technical aspects of these studies as well as on some of the results we obtained so far. Other more clinical and biochemical aspects are discussed elsewhere (2).

Materials and methods

The selection of the patients admitted to the study (62 total, 15 complaining of urological symptoms and 47 visiting our units because of infertility) has been performed as described (2). A sexual abstinence of 7 days, the genocubital position adopted by the patient as well as the slight upward pressure exerced in the pubic region by one of the two clinicians performing the prostatic massage, were of help to obtain the amount of secretion (5−7 drops) needed for cytological, microbiological and electrophoretical analyses [for other details see (2)]. Semen samples were obtained 7−10 days before prostatic massage. The discriminating criteria used for seminal, cytological and microbiological evaluations were as follows: 1. seminal analyses: 0: $<20.10^6$ spermatozoa/ml; A: $<40\%$ progressive motility 2 hrs after ejaculation; T: $<50\%$ normal forms (according to DAVID et al. (3); 2. cytology: <500 (negative), $500−1000$ (doubtful) or >1000 (positive) inflammatory cells/µl of EPS; 3. bacteriology: $<5.10^3$ (negative), $5.10^3−10^4$ (doubtful) or $>10^4$ (positive) aerobic and anaerobic colonies/ml of EPS. The EPS we analysed by electrophoretical of electrofocusing techniques were routinely collected into a 500 µl Eppendorf tube containing 5 µl of a 10 mM solution of PMSF (Serva, West Germany) in isopropanol (8).

This was done to block as much as possible serine proteases before storage of the EPS-samples at $-20°C$. Before electrophoretical analysis the samples were thawed, centrifuged (10 min, 2000 g) and denatured as described below.

Electroanalytical techniques*

All reagent used for SDS-PAGE (A, Bis, SDS, TEMED, β-mercaptoethanol) were from Serva Biochemicals (West Germany) with the exception of Per and Tris which were obtained from Merck (West Germany). Bromophenolblue and Coomassie Blue (R-250 and G-250) were from Fluka (Switzerland). All reagents were of the best available analytical quality. Double, glass-distilled water was used to prepare the A/Bis, SDS, Per and buffer solutions.

The A/Bis solution (28.38 g A/1.62 g Bis per 100 ml) was reprepeared fresh every two−three weeks, filtered and stored in a brown bottle at $+4°C$. Per solution (30 mg/ml) was made fresh every day. Electrophoreses in the presence of SDS were carried out by the Laemmli system (10), using slab-gels of 0.8 mm thickness (5−20% acrylamide gradient). Optimalization and reproducibility of the protein separations were achieved by preparing and running the gels strictly according to the procedure given below. The gel plates ($160 \times 150 \times 0.8$ mm, one with a 23 mm notch) were assembled using hot 1% agar solution and avoiding silicon or other grease type seals. The separation gel was always prepared the day before use by a mini-gradient mixer.

The heavy (T = 20, C = 5.4; A) and light (T = 5.0, C = 5.4; B) solutions were as follows:

---

* *Abbreviations used:* PAGE: polyacrylamide gel electrophoresis, SDS: sodium dodecylsulfate, PAGIEF: polyacrylamide gel isoelectrofocusing, PER: ammonium peroxodisulfate, A: acrylamide, BIS: N, N′-Methylenebisacrylamide, TEMED: N, N, N′, N′-Tetramethylethylenediamine, PMSF: phenylmethyl sulfonylfluoride.

A: 4 ml A/Bis (see above); 1.5 ml of 1.5 M Tris-HCl, pH 8.8; 0.06 ml SDS (10% in H_2O); 0.06 ml Per; 0.38 ml H_2O.

B: 1 ml A/Bis (see above); 1.5 ml of 1.5 M Tris-HCl, pH 8.8; 0.06 ml SDS (10%); 0.06 ml Per and 3.38 ml H_2O.

The total volume was 6.0 ml. Polymerisation was started by adding 3 µl of TEMED to the two solutions in the gradient mixer and elution was started at ~4 ml/min. The gradient surface was immediately covered with 2 ml H_2O (Pasteur pipette) and the gel let to polymerize overnight. Next morning water was removed from the surface of the gel by turning the plates 90° and blotting the inferior edge with filter paper.

The stacking-gel solution [2 ml of A/Bis (see above); 2.5 ml of 0.5 M Tris-HCl, pH 6.8, 0.1 ml SDS (10%), 0.1 ml Per and H_2O to 10 ml, mix, then add 10 µl of TEMED] was poured over the first gel to notch height and immediately a 12- or 20-teeth comb was inserted into the solution. The stacking gel polymerized in 20 min at RT.

Preparation of the samples for electrophoresis

The protein concentration of the samples to be analyzed has to be known exactly: in this study we used with advantage a rapid spectrophotometric method (9), diluting 5 µl of the centrifuged EPS samples (2000 g/10 min/4°C) in 995 l of 0.9% NaCl. Twenty microliters of the sample were mixed in a disposable Eppendorf tube with 20 µl of denaturation buffer [as described in (10)] and 2 µl of β-mercaptoethanol. After vortexing, the well-capped tubes were heated for 10—15 min at 90°C (water bath) then left at RT for about 10 min. The comb was removed from the gel and the pockets filled with SDS-stacking buffer (2.5 ml 0.5 M Tris-HCl pH 6.8 and 0.1 ml 10% SDS to 10 ml with H_2O). Exactly 50 µg protein were then transferred to the gel pockets by the underlayering technique with a 25 µl Hamilton syringe.

Tris-Glycine (electrophoresis) buffer (10) was filled in and 3 drops of 1% bromophenolblue solution (H_2O) added to the upper buffer chamber.

Running and staining conditions

Even careful manipulations in gel preparation resulted in slight variations of the Vo/Io-parameters. Therefore, Vo was always set at 80 V and limited to 200 V (lettiing the mA diminish during the run). Running time was about 3—4 hrs at RT. Staining and destaining was done as described (5) so as to obtain maximal staining (overnight, 1 hr, 1 hr in the 3 solutions).

Results

During preparation of the EPS samples for electrophoresis (denaturation step) a white turbidity was seen to form almost immediately in a number of samples. This turbidity, seldom observed during SDS-denaturation of seminal plasma and probably attribuable to the formation of the sparingly soluble K^+ and/or Ca^{2+} salts of dodecylsulfate [K_{sp} for K^+SDS^- is $1.5.10^{-5}$ (12)] was of no apparent consequence for the stacking or separation of EPS-proteins during SDS-PAGE and disappeared during the run. A screening of all the 62 protein patterns obtained with our gradient slab-gels, showed that 25 of them had an impressive pattern similarity [both in a qualitative (types of proteins) and in a quantitative sense], whereas the other samples presented altered or grossly altered patterns (Fig. 1). Furthermore, by comparing these electrophoretical results with those obtained independently in Magenta (cytology, microbiology) we could observe that there was an interesting coincidence between these "very

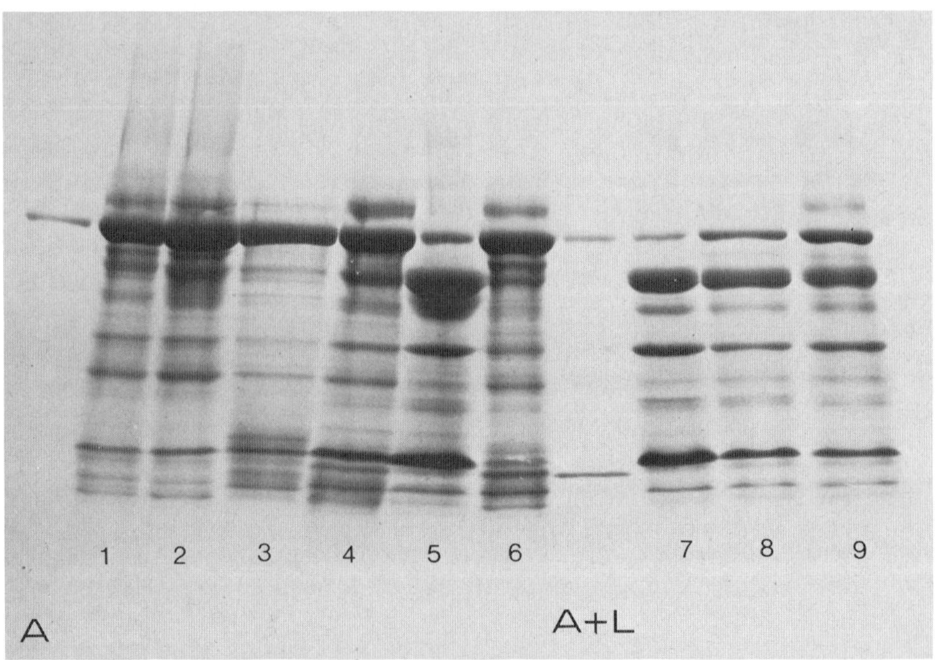

Fig. 1. Electrophoretical analysis of EPS samples obtained from men affected (lanes 1—6) or not affected (lanes 7—9) by prostatic inflammation under denaturing conditions (SDS-PAGE on acrylamide-gradient slab-gels, see Materials and methods for details). The same amount of EPS proteins (50 µg) was run for each sample. Note the striking similarity in the three normal patterns (three different men) and the many differences between them and the "prostatitis" samples. Also note that in many (but not all) samples the concentration of the putative albumin band is strongly augmented. A = albumin, L = lysozym (68 and 14.6 Kdal respectively).

similar protein patterns" and an absence of prostatitis as detected by the two other techniques. All the obtained analytical results are compared in Table 1 and 2, and what we called an "ideal normal EPS-pattern" is shown in Fig. 2 accompanied by the authentical scan of one of these normal (not prostatitis) EPS-samples.

The results obtained by submitting the same EPS-samples to PAGIEF (pH 3−10 gradients) gave analogous results as these obtained by SDS-PAGE: here too prostatitis was accompanied by band-shifts and also by large electroendoosmotic effects [not shown, see (2)].

Unfortunately we were not able to obtain till now a satisfactory resolution of the EPS proteins of our samples with the non-denaturing polyacrylamide gel system Abraham et al. devised for blood proteins (7) and this even in the presence of 0.1% Triton X-100 (Fig. 3). However, even by this unsatisfactory resolution, one can easily observe that the migratory pattern of EPS proteins is

Table 1. Distribution of the studied cases according to the seminological, microbiological and cytological analyses.

| | Prostatitis | | |
	absent*	doubtful*	present*
Various OAT symptoms	17	6	22
Hypospermia	2	0	0
Azoospermia	2	1	1
Normozoospermia	3	2	2
No seminologic data	1	0	3
	25	9	28

* see Table 2.

Tab. 2. Distribution of the studied cases according to electrophoretical, microbiological and cytological analyses.

| | Prostatitis | | |
	absent*	doubtful*	present
Normal protein pattern**	18	2	5
Abnormal protein pattern**	7	7	23
	25	9	28

* According to the results of the microbiological and cytological analyses (discriminating criteria see Materials and methods). The third column (prostatitis present) collects all the cases in which one or both analyses gave a positive result.

** Normal/Abnormal protein pattern defines an EPS protein pattern both qualitatively and quantitatively similar to the "Ideal-normal EPS protein pattern" represented in Fig. 2.

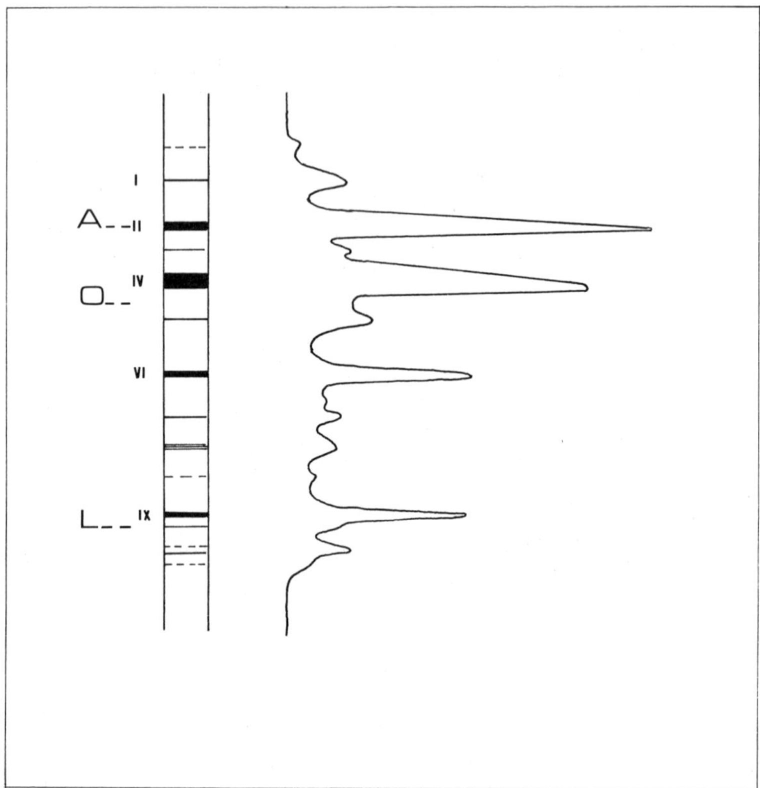

Fig. 2. *Left:* Ideal normal-EPS protein pattern. This pictorial approach gives the approximate positions and intensities (Coomassie coloration) of the major bands of a "non prostatitis" EPS submitted to the gradient SDS-PAGE described in the text and also shown in Fig. 1. A, O, L: albumin (68 Kdal), ovalbumin (45 Kdal) and lysozyme (14.6 Kdal). *Right:* Authentical scan of a "non-prostatitis" (normal) EPS gels pattern.

different from that of blood serum proteins. Of the three major marker-proteins of blood serum (α_2-macroglobulin, transferrin, albumin) only albumin can be easily observed in the EPS gel pattern, although in a much lower concentration (transferrin was seldom observed in such gels, but the presence of protein-protein complexes cannot be ruled out). Discontinuous, non-denaturing gel systems (results not shown) gave even worst results.

Discussion

The results obtained so far [see also (2)] can be considered from a technical, biochemical and clinical point of view. 1. Among all techniques asseyed in this

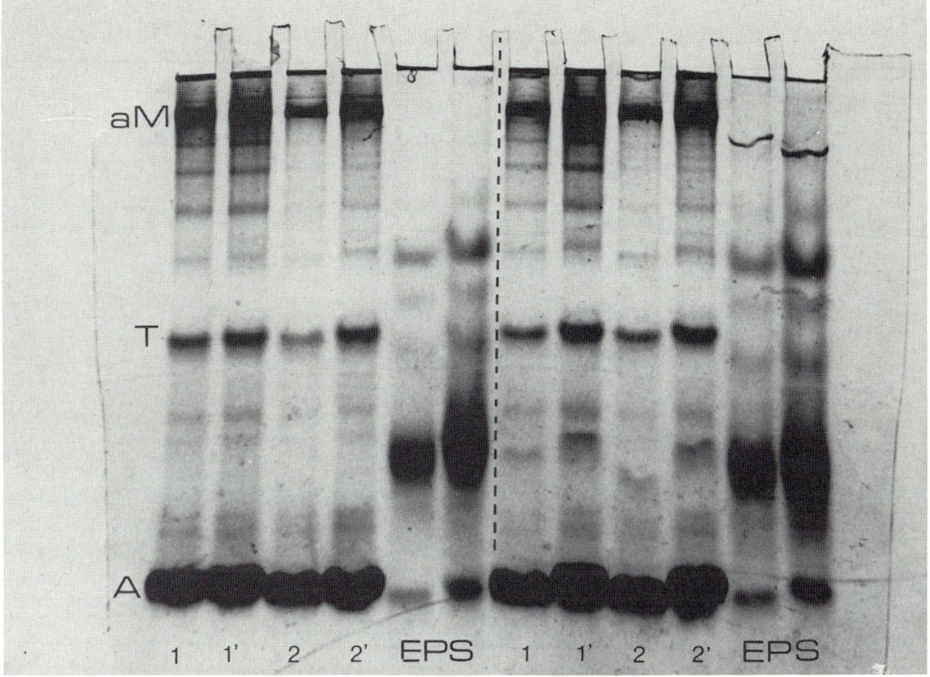

Fig. 3. Non-denaturing electrophoresis of blood and EPS proteins [continuous-buffer, two-gels system of ABRAHAM et al. (7)]. *Left:* 70 (1, 2) and 140 µg (1', 2') of blood serum proteins from two different sera (1, 2) were co-electrophoresed with 30, resp. 60 µg of EPS proteins obtained from a normal man. *Right:* The same samples treated with 0.1% Triton X-100 electrophoresed on the same gel. Glycerol (10% final concentration) was added to all samples for underlayering. aM = α_2-macroglobulin, T = transferrin, A = albumin. Note the lack of resolution of the EPS-samples even in the presence of detergent (ionic-complexes?) as well as the difference in the albumin concentration between blood and prostatic samples.

study, 5–20% acrylamide-gradient SDS-PAGE proved to give the best resolutions of EPS-proteins. 2. It was surprising to find that the protein composition of the secretions obtained from the normal prostates were relatively "simple" and, what is more, extremely similar among different men. The rationale supporting these findings is not clear at present. 3. SDS-PAGE of prostatic secretion was shown in this study to be of clinical interest. Among the 28 men for whom prostatitis was clinically suspected and analytically confirmed (positive cytology and/or microbiology or both), 23 had altered protein patterns. On the contrary, of the 25 patients without prostatitis, 7 were found to have some abnormalities in their EPS-patterns.

We should note that 3 of the 5 normal patterns of the prostatitis group belonged to cases where inflammation was only detected microbiologically (cytology was negative), whereas 5 of the 7 abnormal patterns of the second group (without prostatic inflammation) were found to be associated to a grave dyspermia. Finally, the results of the "doubtful category" probably demonstrates that an SDS-electrophoretical analysis of EPS could be of complementary help in detecting prostatitis for cases where the other analytical data are of insufficient diagnostic value.

Acknowledgement

The present series of studies has been partially supported by the Swiss National Science Foundation and by Hoffman-La Roche (Grants to M. B. and A. C.).

References

(1) BALERNA, M., A. CAMPANA, D. FABBRO, U. EPPENBERGER: High-resolution seminal plasma protein patterns in normal and infertile men. In: HAFEZ, E. S. E., K. SEMM (eds.): Instrumental Insemination; pp. 17−25. Martinus Nijhoff, The Hague 1982.

(2) BALERNA, M., G. M. COLPI, A. CAMPANA, L. ROVEDA, A. TOMMASINI-DEGNA, A. ZANOLLO: High-resolution protein patterns of human expressed prostatic secretion: A new tool for the diagnosis of prostatitis. Arch. Andrology 8: 97−105 (1982).

(3) DAVID, G., J. P. BISSON, P. JOUANNET, S. CZYGLIK, C. GERNINON, C. ALEXANDRE, C. GILBERT-DREYFUS: Les Tératospermies. In: THIBAULT, C. (eds.): Fecundité et Sterilité du mâle; pp. 81−102. Masson, Paris 1972.

(4) ELIASSON, R.: Oxygen consumption of human spermatozoa in seminal plasma and a Ringer solution. J. Reprod. Fertil. 27: 385−389 (1971).

(5) FAIRBANKS, G., T. L. STECK, D. F. H. WALLACH: Electrophoretic analysis of the major polypeptides of the human erythrocyte membrane. Biochemistry. 10: 2606−2616 (1971).

(6) HOFFMANN, N., L. WILSCH: Störungen der männlichen Fertilität bei unspezifischen chronischen Entzündungen der akzessorischen Geschlechtsdrüsen. Therapiewoche 19: 1700−1706 (1973).

(7) ABRAHAM, K., K. SCHUETT, I. MUELLER, H. HOFFMEISTER: Kontinuierliche Polyacrylamid-Elektrophorese. II. Untersuchungen an Normalseren. Z. klin. Chem. klin. Biochem. 8: 92−98 (1970).

(8) JAMES, G. T.: Inactivation of the protease inhibitor Phenylmethylsulfonyl fluoride in buffers. Anal. Biochem. 86: 574−579 (1978).

(9) KALB, V. F., R. W. BERNLOHR: A new spectrophotometric assay for proteins in cell extracts. Anal. Biochem. 82: 362−371 (1977).

(10) LAEMMLI, U. K., M. FAVRE: Maturation of the head of bacteriophage T_4. I: DNA packing events. J. Mol. Biol. 80: 575−599 (1973).

(11) LINDHOLMER, CH.: The importance of seminal plasma for human sperm motility. Fertil. Steril. 10: 533−542 (1974).

(12) NEMAN, R. L.: Dodecyl Sodium Sulphate as a reagent for the detection of potassium. J. Chem. Educ. 44: 479−481 (1967).

(13) OVERSTREET, J. M., C. COATS, D. F. KATZ, F. W. HANSON: The importance of seminal plasma for sperm penetration of human cervical mucus. Fertil. Steril. 34: 569−572 (1980).

(14) TRIFUNAC, N. P., G. S. BERNSTEIN: Inhibition of the oxidative metabolism of human spermatozoa by a heat-labile factor in seminal plasma. Fertil. Steril. 27: 1295−1300 (1976).

(15) YOUNG, L. G., S. A. GOODMAN: Characterization of human sperm cell surface components. Biol. Reprod. 23: 826−835 (1980).

*Urologische Klinik der Universität München (Direktor: Prof. Dr. E. Schmiedt),
Klinikum Großhadern, München*

Biochemical Analysis of Prostatic Fluid in Chronic Inflammation: pH, Immunoglobulins and Proteins*

H. W. Bauer, W. Sturm, J. Schüller, E. Schmiedt

Introduction

Due to the apocrine mechanism of secretion, in which the granules are secreted with inclusion of cytoplasm portions of the prostate gland cells, prostate secretion is the most representative starting material in order to study alterations in the prostate. The ejaculate is more readily accessible and is available in larger amounts, but the prostate secretion undergoes changes which no longer permit any relevant inferences due to admixtures from the seminal vesicles, the bulbourethral glands and the spermatozoa. Thus the plasma proteins and immunoglobulins in the ejaculate are noticeably reduced compared to the prostatic fluid. Spermatozoa can be loaded, for example, with portions of the immunoglobulin fraction either purely adsorptively or (probably more rarely) by immunological cross-reactions.

Alterations with regard to the cell number (Bourne and Frishette, 1967), the bacteriological findings (Meares, 1968), the pH value (Ludvik, 1964) and the protein content (Soanes et al., 1961) of the prostatic fluid in the context of chronic inflammatory processes of the prostate have been known for a long time. The alterations are so severe that one can even refer to a general secretory dysfunction of the prostate.

There is no doubt that these secretory dysfunctions have great influence also on the penetration of antimicrobial substances into the prostate.

pH value

The simplest parameter indicating alterations of the prostate secretion is the pH value. In the studies of Huggins et al. (1942), a pH value of 6.4 to 6.5 was still regarded as a fixed parameter. However, the studies of Blacklock and

* Supported by the Deutsche Forschungsgemeinschaft, Bonn-Bad Godesberg (Ba 706/1).

BEAVIS (1974), ANDERSON and FAIR (1976), PFAU et al. (1978) as well as COR-
DONNIER (1979) have given rise to uncertainty with regard to this so far undis-
puted parameter.

BLACKLOCK and BEAVIS found that the pH value in a normal man is around
6.6. ANDERSON and FAIR reported values around 7.6, PFAU a pH value around
6.7, FAIR and CORDONNIER a pH value around 7.28.

We found an average pH value of 7.15 in 36 patients without indications of
an acute or chronic inflammatory process in the male adnexa. In accordance
with a stratification according to age, it is shown that the pH value is displaced
with increasing age from the weakly acid to the weakly alkaline range. These
results are consistent with the data of FAIR and CORDONNIER from 1979.

We have carried out the pH measurements with a microelectrode of a pH
meter. The calibration is accurate to one decimal place of the pH (Fig. 1).

Irrespective of the discrepancy of the pH value of the prostatic fluid in
healthy men, all investigators have in common that they found a weakly alkaline prostatic fluid pH in patients with chronic prostatitis. This value was also
at 7.8 with a simple standard deviation of 0.5 in our investigations. These
results are more significant, since a diffusion of the antibiotic along the pH
gradient is desired in antimicrobial therapy (WININGHAM, NEMOY and STAMEY,
1968).

Organic anions, especially citrate and proteins, are responsible for the ionic
equilibrium in the prostatic fluid. Besides the reduction of the citric acid (FAIR

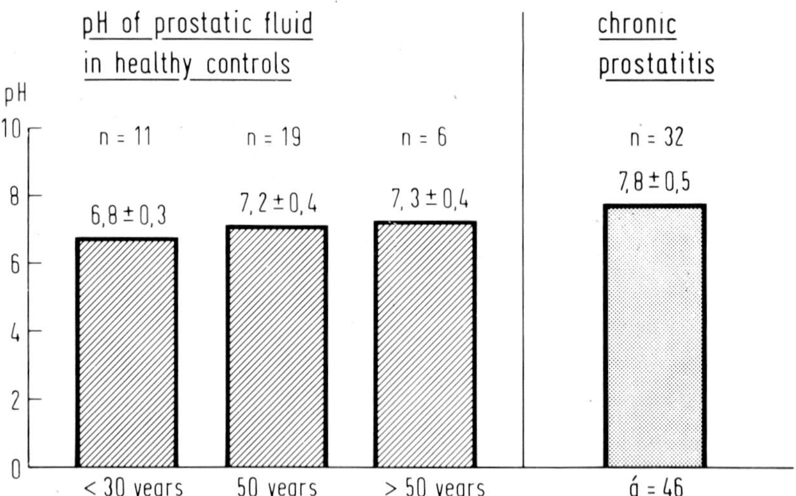

Fig. 1. pH values in prostatic fluid in test subjects without clinical indications of an acute or
chronic inflammatory process in the male adnexa (n = 36) and in patients with chronic prostatitis
(n = 32).

and CORDONNIER, 1978) in the prostatic fluid in chronic prostatitis, the altered immunoglobulin content in chronic prostatitis appears to be responsible for the alteration of the pH value in the direction of basicity. With a total protein content of 2 g/dl, about 5% of the proteins are immunoglobulins.

Immunoglobulins

The first determinations of immunoglobulins in the prostate secretion derived from CHODIRKER and TOMASI (1963). Alterations of immunoglobulin concentration in the prostatic fluid have been demonstrated again and again in the subsequent years, e. g. by BREHM and LACHNER (1968) and GRAY et al. (1974), although no normal values were available from representative subjects.

We first of all investigated the immunoglobulins IgG, IgA, IgM of 25 healthy subjects of varying age with an urological anamnesis which had been normal so far. We found the following concentrations (see Fig. 2): for IgM, the primary reactant of the humoral immune response, we found a mean concentration of 7 mg/dl, for immunoglobulin G, the main representative of the immuno-globulins and secondary reactants with an appreciably longer residence time and higher concentrations, we found mean secretion concentrations of 30 mg/dl; the simple standard deviation was 7.5 mg/dl. The mucoprotectant representatives of the immunoglobulin class, IgA, showed mean concentrations around 12 mg/dl at 3 mg/dl standard deviation.

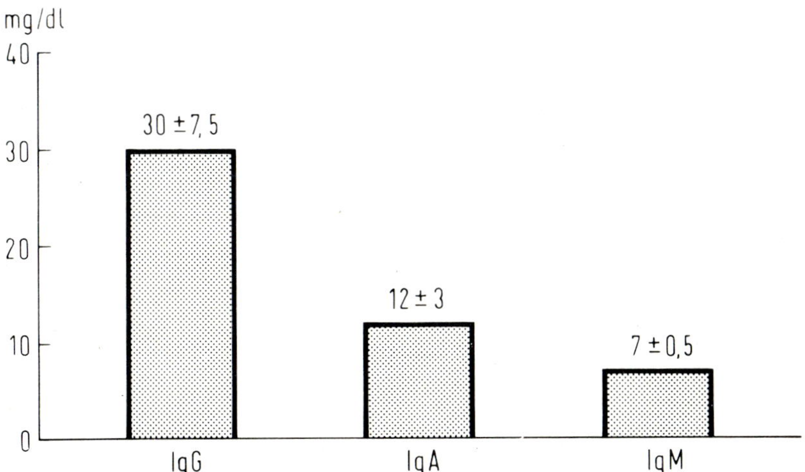

Fig. 2. Concentration of immunoglobulins IgG, IgA, IgM in prostatic fluid in healthy test subjects of different ages (n = 25).

Comparison of these results for immunoglobulin concentrations which we found in prostatic fluid in 60 patients with chronic prostatitis shows distinct increases in concentration, especially for IgG and IgA (Fig. 3).

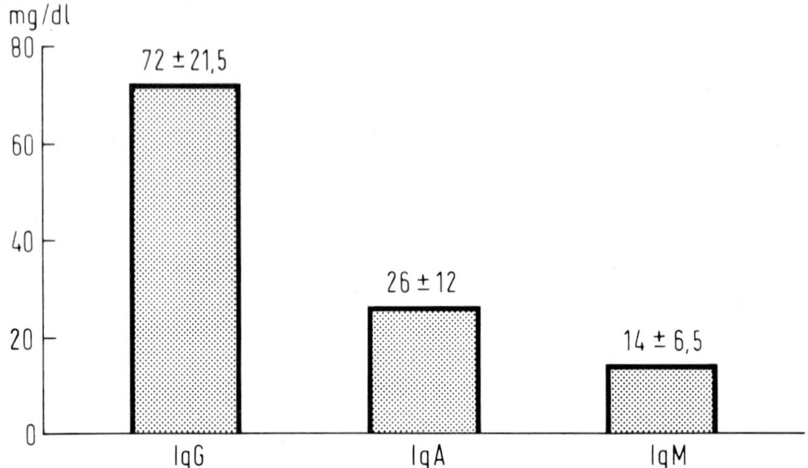

Fig. 3. Concentration of immunoglobulins IgG, IgA, IgM in prostatic fluid in patients with chronic prostatitis (n = 60).

The even higher immunoglobulin concentrations in the study of GRAY et al. (1974) are probably to be explained in that we have only rarely obtained prostatic fluid around the peak of the clinical symptoms. On the other hand, we believe that we can document a certain methodological progress due to nephelometric determination of the immunoglobulins (BAUER et al., 1980). The relatively high standard deviations in the immunoglobulins G and A can be interpreted in terms of a trend to two different groups with regard to the immunoglobulin classes IgG and IgA. The one group with more or less continuously high values of IgG and IgA and one group in which the concentrations decreased during treatment (whether post or propter). The unchanged IgM concentrations in our study group must likewise be interpreted in that the determination took place immediately at the beginning of the symptom-peak in a few cases only.

"Acute-phase" proteins

The experience that the alpha glycoproteins increase rapidly and intensively in acute infections, in inflammations, but also in necrotizing processes has led to combination of these plasma proteins under the overall term "acute-phase" proteins.

A proportion of these proteins was already determined qualitatively in the paper by LENNERT and SCHRÖDER (1970). In particular, ceruloplasmin and the complement component C3c were considered significant in differential diagnosis between inflammatory and noninflammatory adnex-diseases in the studies of BLENK et al. (1974) as well as KRAUSE and WEIDNER (1978). However, this was contradicted by other authors (NEUMANN and MAUSS, 1978). Our results (Fig. 4 and 5) show a clear difference of concentration of the "acute-phase" proteins haptoglobin, alpha$_2$ macroglobulin, acid alpha$_1$ glycoprotein and ceruloplasmin between healthy subjects and patients with an acute episode of chronic prostatitis.

Whereas the elevation of the "acute-phase" proteins can be explained as the consequence of an increased vascular permeability in the context of inflammatory manifestations, an increased local regional synthesis must also be considered in the case of the immunoglobulins. The local regional lymph nodes may be responsible for this. This is indicated also by the results of TOMASI and ZIGLBAUM (1963). They show that the specific antibody is more highly concentrated in the gland cell of the prostate than in the periphery.

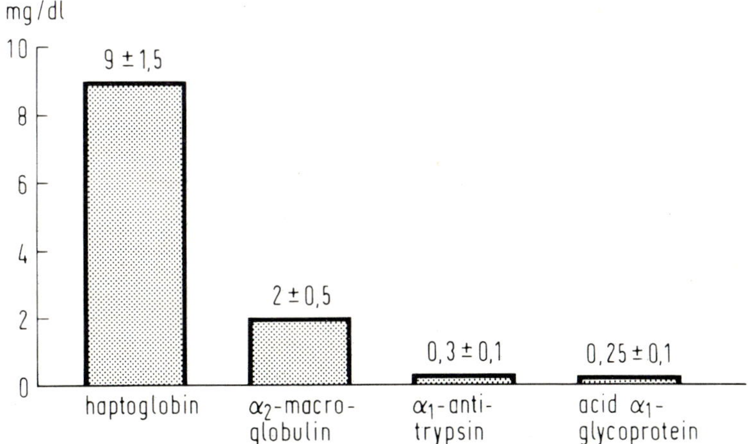

Fig. 4. Concentration of "acute-phase" proteins haptoglobin, alpha$_2$ macroglobulin, alpha$_1$ antitrypsin, acid alpha$_1$ glycoprotein in prostatic fluid in healthy subjects (n = 25).

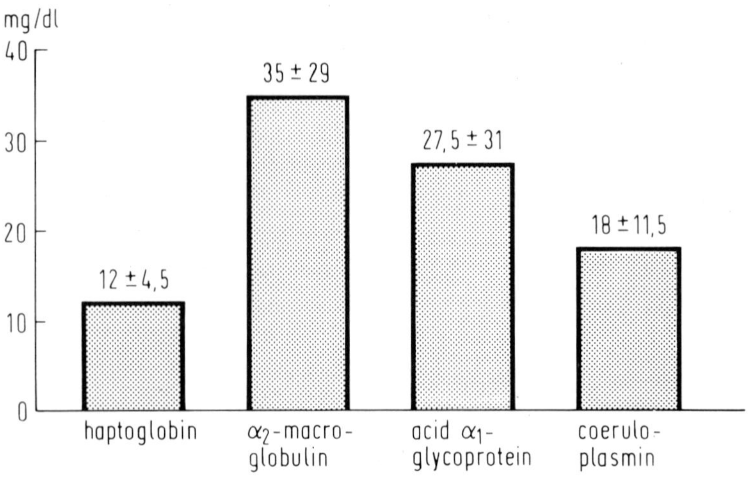

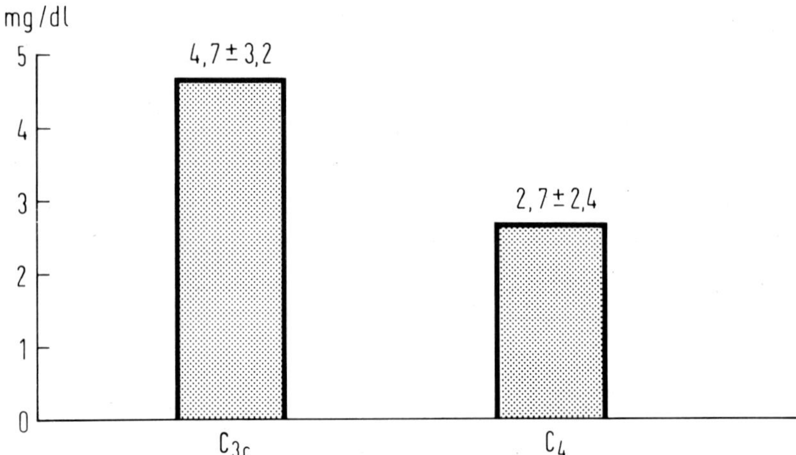

Fig. 5. *Above:* Concentration of "acute-phase" proteins haptoglobin, alpha₂ macroglobulin, alpha₁ antitrypsin, acid alpha₁ glycoprotein in prostatic fluid in patients with an acute episode of chronic prostatitis (n = 15) and *below:* of complement C3c and C4 (n = 27).

Summary

Alterations of the pH value and the concentration of immunoglobulins and "acute-phase" proteins are manifestations of a general secretory dysfunction of the prostate in chronic prostatitis. Demonstration of altered immunoglobulins and "acute-phase" protein concentrations in prostatic fluid can thus contribute to differentiation of inflammatory processes from autonomic urogenital syndromes. However, the future diagnosis of inflammatory processes in the prostate will not take place via determination of total globulins, but by means of specific antibodies.

References

(1) ANDERSON, R. N., W. R. FAIR: Physical and chemical determinations of prostatic secretion in benign hyperplasia, prostatitis and adenocarcinoma. Invest. Urol. *14*: 137−140 (1976).

(2) BAUER, H. W., P. MAYER, H. E. MELLIN, J. SCHÜLLER, F. J. MARX: Lasernephelometrischer Nachweis von Immunglobulinen und „Akute Phase" Proteinen im Prostataexprimat und Ejakulat bei entzündlichen Adnexprozessen. Verhandlungsbericht der Dt. Gesellschaft für Urologie XXXI. S. 35−36, 1980.

(3) BLACKLOCK, N. J., J. P. BEAVIS: The response of prostatic fluid pH in inflammation. Brit. J. Urol. *46*: 537−541 (1974).

(4) BLENK, H., A. HOFSTETTER, R. BOWERING, R. BUTTLER, M. HARTMANN, F. J. MARX: Immunelektrophorese des Ejakulats. Münch. med. Wschr. *106*: 35−38 (1974).

(5) BOURNE, C. W., W. A. FRISHETTE: Prostatic fluid analysis and prostatosis. J. Urol. *97*: 140−143 (1967).

(6) BREHM, G., H. LACHNER: Quantitative Immunglobulinbestimmungen im Seminalplasma. Klin. Wschr. *46*: 902−904 (1968).

(7) CHODIRKER, W. B., T. B. TOMASI: Gamma-globulins: Quantitative relationship in human semen and nonvascular fluids. Science *142*: 1080−1083 (1963).

(8) FAIR, W. R., J. J. CORDONNIER: The pH of prostatic fluid: a reappraisal and therapeutic implications. J. Urol. *120*: 695−697 (1979).

(9) GRAY, S. P., J. BILLINGS, N. J. BLACKLOCK: Distribution of the immunglobulins A and M in the prostatic fluid of patients with prostatitis. Clin. Chim. Acta *57*: 163−166 (1974).

(10) HUGGINS, C., W. W. SCOTT, J. H. HEINEN: Chemical composition of human semen and of secretion of prostate and seminal vesicles. Amer. J. Physiol. *136*: 467−469 (1942).

(11) KRAUSE, W., W. WEIDNER: Proteinkonzentrationen im Ejakulat bei Patienten mit chronischer Prostatitis. Hautarzt *29*: 648−649 (1978).

(12) LENNERT, K. A., H. M. SCHRÖDER: Immunologische Untersuchungen der Serumproteine im Prostataexprimat. Münch. med. Wschr. *25*: 1224−1227 (1970).

(13) LUDVIK, W.: Zur Diagnostik der chronischen Prostatitis. Dtsch. med. Wschr. *89*: 2366−2369 (1964).

(14) MEARES, E. M., F. A. STAMEY: Bacteriologic localization patterns in bacterial prostatitis and urethritis. Invest. Urol. *5*: 492−493 (1968).

(15) NEUMANN, R., J. MAUSS: Die Bedeutung der Bestimmung von C3c Komplement und Coeruloplasmin für den Nachweis einer Infektion im Bereich der samenableitenden Wege. Hautarzt *29*: 383−385 (1978).

(16) PFAU, A., S. PERLBERG, A. SHAPIRA: The pH of prostatic fluid in health and disease: implications of treatment in chronic bacterial prostatitis. J. Urol. *119*: 384−388 (1978).

(17) Shortliff, L. M. D., U. Wehner, Th. A. Stamey: The detection of local prostatic immunologic response to bacterial prostatitis. J. Urol. *125*: 509 (1981).
(18) Soanes, W. A., E. R. Gabrielli, K. H. Felch: Biochemical classification of prostatitis: based on electrophoretic study of prostatic fluid. J. Urol. *85*: 621–623 (1961).
(19) Winnigham, D. G., N. J. Nemoy, T. A. Stamey: Diffusion of antibiotics from plasma into prostatic fluid. Nature *219*: 139–142 (1968).

Institut für Wehrmedizin und Hygiene, Ernst-Rodenwaldt-Institut, Koblenz
(Direktor: Oberstarzt Dr. med. H. Blenk)
Urologische Klinik der Medizinischen Hochschule Lübeck (Direktor: Prof. Dr. A. Hofstetter)

The Behaviour of Complement C3 and other Serum Proteins in the Ejaculate in Chronic Prostatitis and their Diagnostic Importance

H. BLENK, A. HOFSTETTER

Normally, the occurrence of acute prostatitis and prostato-adnexitis is accompanied by a pronounced clinical symptomatology and a considerable increase of leucocytes and high cell counts in the prostata-exprimate or ejaculate. Thus, from the diagnostic point of view, this presents hardly any problem. Chronic prostatitis, however, is an altogether different matter.

In addition to the often non-specific clinical symptomatology and the difficulty to demonstrate the presence of relevant bacteria (SCHNIERSTEIN, 1974; MEARES, 1980), earlier assumptions could not be verified, namely that in the exprimate of patients with chronic prostatitis, in contrast to healthy people, always more than 20 leucocytes are observed per 400× power field. When examining 311 *healthy* males, O'SHAUGNESSY, PARRINO and WHITE (1956) found that about 30% of the test persons had over 50 leucocytes per 400× power field. SCHNIERSTEIN (1964 and 1965) confirmed these results by means of tests conducted with Federal Armed Forces military personnel. Therefore, LUDVIK (1964) suggested an exact quantitative count of leucocytes in the prostatic secretion. As the upper normal value in a healthy person, LUDVIK found 300,000 leucocytes per ml prostatic secretion, while in cases of inflammation more than 3×10^5 and up to 5 million leucocytes are detected. Although this quantitative counting method is considered to be rather reliable, it is very time-consuming and can only be used for the prostatic secretion. Due to the small quantity of prostate exprimate obtainable in most cases it is, however, not very suitable to be transported to a qualified microbiological laboratory, on which many urologists have to depend. The ejaculate is better suited for transportation to the laboratory; however, the quantitative leucocyte count cannot be precisely evaluated due to the high proportion of sperm and cells from spermiogenesis. Therefore, it was considered whether other parameters such as immunoglobulins or acute-phase-proteins would not be better suited for the evaluation of the inflammatory activity in the male adnexa.

Albumin
α-1-Antitrypsin
Saures -α1-
Glycoprotein
J. g. G.
Komplement C 3
Transferrin
Haptoglobin

Fig. 1a.

Saures-α1-
Glycoprotein
Albumin
α-1-Antitrypsin
Transferrin
J. g. G.

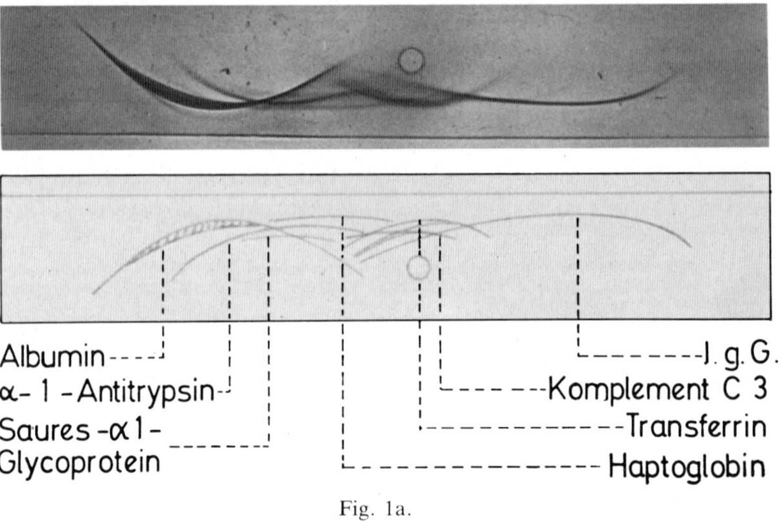

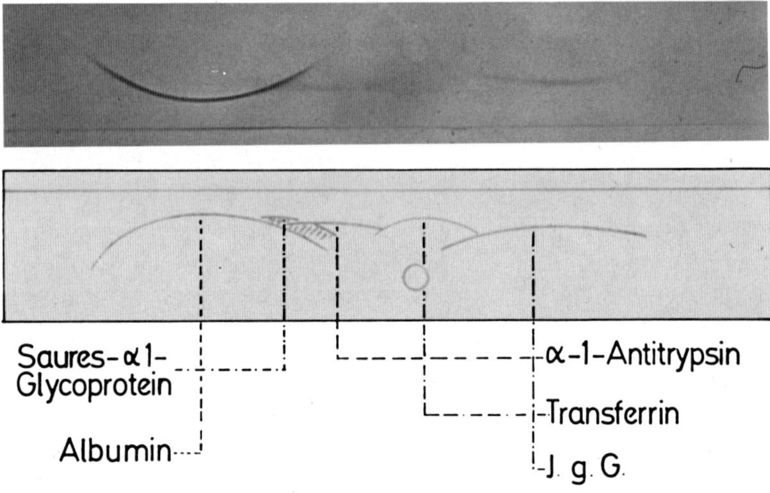

Fig. 1b.

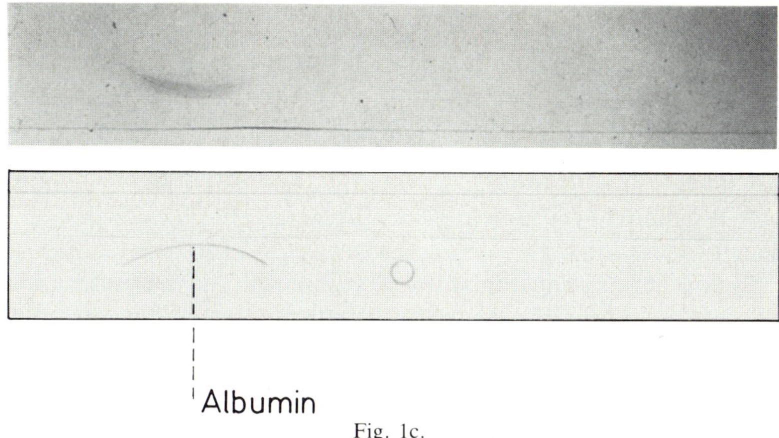

Fig. 1c.

Fig. 1. Immunelectrophoreses of the ejaculate from a patient with acute prostatitis (a) chronic prostatitis (b), a healthy man respectively from a patient with vegetative urogenital syndrome (c). The number of bands documents the distinctions between the different degrees of inflammation compared with healthy persons resp. patients with vegetative urogenital syndrome (VUG).

Studies regarding the concentrations of immunoglobulin A, G and M in the prostate-experimate had shown that in cases of acute and chronic prostatitis 50% to 70% of the patients had higher immunoglobulin levels than healthy persons (HEREMANNS, 1960; BARNES et al., 1963; LENNERT, 1970; JONAS and HÖVENER, 1973). Our immuno-electrophoretic studies with ejaculate and also quantitative analyses of immunoglobulins and serumproteins not only led to corresponding results but also showed that in the case of prostatitis not only the immunoglobulins had increased but also other protein fractions (Fig. 1a–c) (BLENK et al., 1974a).

For this reason, a clinical-microbiological study under controlled conditions was conducted involving 131 males between 18 and 50 years, affected by various diseases of the urogenital tract due to infectuous-inflammatory processes and psychogenic alterations. For control purposes, these cases were compared with 30 healthy males (BLENK et al., 1974b; BLENK and HOFSTETTER, 1975).

In addition to the detailed anamnestic and clinical urological exploration, a microscopic (including quantitative leucocyte count) and microbiological examination of midstream urine, prostate exprimate, exprimate urine and ejaculate was conducted. Following a perineal biopsy of the prostate, performed with the TRI-CUT-needle, an additional histopathologic examination of the prostate tissue was conducted with 50 of these patients in order to substantiate the clinical and laboratory findings by means of an additional method for a part of the cases.

Considering these conditions, the following diagnoses were made for the 131 patients:

Solitary urethritis	= 14 patients	5 biopsies
Chronic adnexitis	= 43 patients	23 biopsies
Acute urethro-adnexitis	= 30 patients	5 biopsies
Chronic and acute epididymitis	= 11 patients	2 biopsies
Vegetative urogenital syndrome ("Psychogenic Prostatitis")	= 33 patients	15 biopsies

According to the findings obtained from clinical and laboratory examinations, all (30) voluntary and healthy test persons were free of pathological findings.

These diagnoses were compared with results of the quantitative determination of different protein fractions (radial immune diffusion according to MANCINI) of the ejaculates of both the patients as well as the healthy persons.

The results (Table 1) show that the presence of some proteins such as complement C3, coeruloplasmin, alpha-2-macroglobulin and haptoglobin in the ejaculate of healthy persons as well as in patients with solitary urethritis and vegetative urogenital syndrome could not be demonstrated at all or only in very minute quantities (less than 0.005 g/l).

Table 1. Level of the mean values of the different protein fractions (given in g/l) of the ejaculate of healthy persons as well as of patients with the vegetative urogenital syndrome "Psychogenic Prostatitis" and inflammatory diseases of the male adnexa and epididymis.

Protein fraction	Healthy control	Vegetative urogenital syndrome	Solitary urethritis	Chronic adnexitis and epididymitis	Acute adnexitis and epididymitis
Albumin	0.59	0.63	0.69	1.6	4.7
Acid-α-1-glycoprotein	0.03	0.03	0.03	0.1	0.25
α-1-antitrypsin	0.08	0.07	0.08	0.12	0.22
Coeruloplasmin	0	0	0	0.0075	0.05
Haptoglobin	0	0	0	0.009	0.14
α-2-macroglobulin	0	0	0	0.007	0.12
Complement C3c	0.005	0.005	0.005	0.04	0.12
Transferrin	0.04	0.04	0.05	0.11	0.28
IgA	0.02	0.01	0.03	0.13	0.35
IgG	0.21	0.21	0.22	0.49	2.40

Other proteins such as albumin, alpha-1-antitrypsin, acid-alpha-1-glycoprotein, transferrin as well as IgA and IgG were found in small quantities in the ejaculate of the healthy persons as well as of the patients with urethritis and

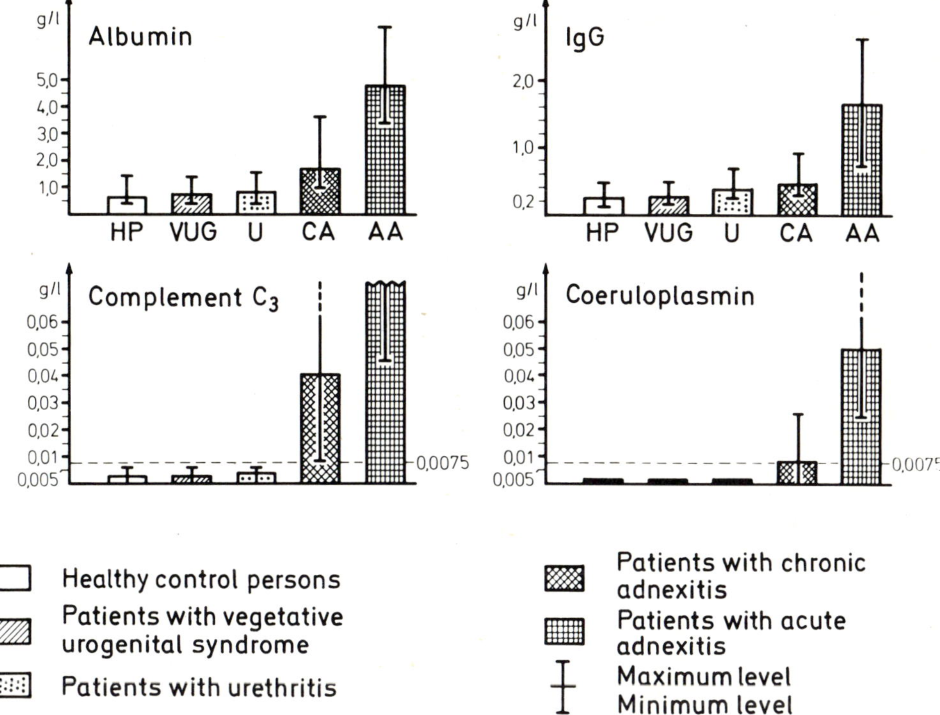

Fig. 2. Levels of albumin, IgG, complement C3 and coeruloplasmin in relation to the two different groups of patients and urogenital diseases.

vegetative urogenital syndrome. As far as patients with chronic inflammations are concerned, a rise in the level of C3, IgG, IgA, transferrin, alpha-1-antitrypsin, alpha-1-glycoprotein, and albumin is apparent with *all* patients, whereas only 30% to 50% of the patients had higher levels of coeruloplasmin, haptoglobin and alpha-2-macroglobulin. In cases of acute prostatitis (adnexitis) and epididymitis, all protein fractions measured in the ejaculate showed a significant rise.

The results of this examination may be summarized as follows (Fig. 2):

a) Concentrations exceeding 0.005 g/l of complement fraction C3 can be found in the ejaculate only in cases of chronic and acute inflammation of the male adnexa.

b) In only 37% of the cases with chronic inflammatory adnexa diseases can coeruloplasmin be found in the ejaculate in concentrations exceeding 0.005 g/l, whereas this margin was exceeded in all cases with acute adnexitis.

Table 2. Comparison of results from clinical, microbiological (exclusive of Chlamydia) and histological findings with the behaviour of the levels of complement, coeruloplasmin and IgG in the ejaculate of patients suffering from chronic adnexitis and vegetative urogenital syndrome.

Item No.	Clinical Diagnosis	Subjective complaints	Clinical findings	Prostate exprimate leucocytes	bacteria count
1	Solitary urethritis	+	+	0.8×10^5	Ø
2	Acute exacerbated adnexitis	+	+	10^6	Enterococci 10^4
3	Chronic adnexitis	+	+	1.5×10^5	Staph. aureus 4×10^3
4	Chronic adnexitis	+	Without pathological findings	2.8×10^5	Ø
5	Chronic recurrent adnexitis	+	Without pathological findings	8×10^6	Ø
6	Adnexitis	+	Without pathological findings	2.5×10^6	Ø
7	Prostate adenoma	+	+	8×10^5	Enterococci 7×10^3
8	Chronic adnexitis	+	Without pathological findings	1.8×10^5	Ø
9	Chronic adnexitis	+	+	10^6	Staph. aureus 3×10^3
10	Chronic recurrent urethro-adnexitis	+	Without pathological findings	1.5×10^6	U. urealyticum 10^4
11	Chronic adnexitis	+	+	1.3×10^6	Staph. aureus 5×10^3
12	Chronic adnexitis and epididymitis	+	+	3.2×10^5	Ø
13	Vegetative urogenital syndrome	+	Without pathological findings	0.8×10^5	Ø
14	Vegetative urogenital syndrome	+	+	3.5×10^5	Enterococci 10^3
15	Vegetative urogenital syndrome	+	+	3.2×10^5	Ø
16	Vegetative urogenital syndrome	+	+	10^5	Ø

Table 2 (continued).

midstream urine leucocytes/ ($\times$ 1000)	bacteria count	Histological findings	Complement C3	Coeruloplasmin	IgG
20	M. hominis 10^3	Normal prostate tissue	0.005	Ø	0.28
1−2	Ø	Serious chronic lymphocytic inflammation	0.18	0.6	1.97
Ø	Ø	Chronic fibrous leucocytic inflammation	0.04	0.0075	0.79
1−3	Ø	Chronic fibrous inflammation	0.0075	Ø	0.26
3−5	Ø	Serious leucocytic and lymphocytic focal inflammation	0.12	0.05	0.76
3−5	Ø	Focal, chronic degenerative inflammation	0.03	Ø	0.56
1	Ø	Increased fibromuscular stroma and chronic leucocytic inflammation	0.08	Ø	0.23
Ø	Ø	Slight inflammatory changes	0.0075	Ø	0.39
Ø	Ø	Low-level leucocytic infiltrate	0.0075	Ø	0.31
40−50	U. urealyticum 5×10^3 Staph. aureus 4×10^2	Lymphocytic and leucocytic inflammation, fibroses	0.04	Ø	0.39
5−7	Ø	Serious focal plasmacytic, lymphocytic degenerative inflammation	0.06	0.02	0.59
Ø	Ø	1. Chronic fibrous inflammation 2. Chronic leucocytic fibrous epididymitis	0.04	0.03	0.59
Ø	Ø	Normal prostate tissue	Ø	Ø	0.16
Ø	Ø	Normal prostate tissue	0.005	Ø	0.23
Ø	Ø	Normal prostate tissue	0.005	Ø	0.19
Ø	Ø	Normal prostate tissue	0.005	Ø	0.19

c) The level of both proteins in the ejaculate, in particular that of the coeruloplasmin, correlates with the degree of the inflammation, that is, it provides a
parameter for the degree of the inflammatory activity.

d) In cases of solitary urethritis, neither C3 nor coeruloplasmin can be found in
the ejaculates, allowing to differentiate between urethritis and adnexitis
patients.

e) As far as psychogenic complaints pertaining to the urogenital tract are concerned (e. g. vegetative urogenital syndrome), the level of C3 or coeruloplasmin, resp. in the ejaculate lies below 0.005 g/l. Thus, one is able to differentiate between such syndromes and inflammatory processes.

Therefore, for the quantitative determination of complement C3 and
coeruloplasmin in the ejaculate, the following margins were established for
assessment purposes:

Complement C3: up to 0.005 g/l = standard;
                0.0075 g/l = indication of adnexitis
Coeruloplasmin: up to 0.005 g/l = standard;
                0.0075 g/l = indication of adnexitis

f) As regards the other protein fractions in the ejaculate, including immunoglobulins A and G, the levels found in patients with chronic adnexitis were in
part below the maximum levels found in healthy persons, thus, no upper
standard level can be clearly determined for these proteins.

By means of 16 selected and biopsied patients, the diverging statements of
the different parameters used in this study are illustrated in Table 2.

On the other hand, this table also reflects concurrence between the histology
and the C3-determinations. Only in one case (2%) of the biopsied patients the
histopathologic finding (normal prostate tissue) did not concur with the slightly
positive level of C3 (0.0075 g/l). Thus, a very high reliability with respect to the
determination of C3 in the ejaculate can be expected concerning the identification of an inflammatory process of the adnexa.

The cause for the increase of the complement in the ejaculate in cases of
infection of the male adnexa is to be understood, in the process of the inflammatory reaction, as a consequence of the immune response to the microorganisms and their catabolite products (AUSTIN and COHN, 1963). As regards the
effectiveness of the immune reaction, the complement system, in cooperation
with the antibodies, is essential for opsonization, phagocytosis and "killing" of
the microorganisms (ATKINSON and FRANK, 1980; ROITT, 1977). The effectiveness of the protection provided by the humoral antibodies depends on the
functional effectiveness of this complement-phagocytosis system since the killing effect of the antibodies with respect to an infectuous microorganism is
determined by the amplifying function of these systems (KOHLER, 1978; SOMER
et al., 1980).

The antigen-antibody-reaction induces a complement activation and leads to the release of chemotactical and anaphylactic substances leading subsequently to an increased vascular permeability as well as exudation of inflammatory cells and plasma proteins and thus, also of C3 (SELL, 1977; SOMER et al., 1980). This explains not only the rise of the serum protein level (i. a. also that of C3, IgG and coeruloplasmin) in the ejaculate in cases of acute adnexitis but also the decrease of IgG and coeruloplasmin to the standard level, if the inflammatory process is barely active and when the increased permeability is no longer present.

In contrast to the decrease of IgG and coeruloplasmin, the persistent multiplication of the complement in case of a barely active chronic adnexitis could only be explained by the complement production of macrophages (COLTON, 1974 and 1977 as cited by ATKINSON and FRANK, 1980; Miller 1981).

With macro- (and already micro-)hemato-spermia, a meaningful statement concerning an inflammatory process of the adnexa cannot be made on the basis of these parameters since a hemorrhage in the area of the prostate or the appending organs allows plasma proteins − among them C3 and coeruloplasmin − to enter into the ejaculate in addition to erythrocytes. By carefully microscoping the ejaculate, the presence of erythrocytes (>1 erythrocyte per field of view $\times 1000$) has first to be excluded.

References

(1) ATKINSON, J. P., M. M. FRANK: Complement. In: PARKER, CH. W. (ed.): Clinical Immunology, p. 219. W. B. Saunders, Philadelphia−London−Toronto 1980.

(2) AUSTIN, K. F., Z. A. COHN: Contribution of serum and cellular factors in host defense reactions. New Engl. J. Med. 268: 933 (1963).

(3) BARNES, G. W., W. A. SOANES, L. MARNROD, M. J. GONDER, S. SHULMAN: Immunologic properties of human prostatic fluid. J. Lab. clin. Med. 61: 578 (1963).

(4) BLENK, H., B. BRAUN, A. HOFSTETTER: Abgrenzung vegetativer Störungen von entzündlichen Prozessen im Bereich der männlichen Adnexe durch immunologisches Verfahren. Wehrmed. Mschr. 3: 79 (1974a).

(5) BLENK, H., A. HOFSTETTER, R. BÖWERING, R. BUTTLER, M. HARTMANN, F. J. MARX: Immunelektrophorese des Ejakulates. Münch. med. Wschr. 116: 35 (1974b).

(6) BLENK, H., A. HOFSTETTER: Quantitative Eiweißanalyse des Ejakulates. Lab. Blätter 25: 166 (1975).

(7) COLTEN, H. R.: Complement synthesis. In: GOOD, R. A., S. B. DAY, (eds.): Comprehensive Immunology 2. Biological Amplification System in Immunology, p. 47. Plenum Publishing Co., New York 1977 [zit. b. (1)].

(8) COLTEN, H. R.: Synthesis and metabolism of complement proteins. Transplant Proc. 6: 33 (1974) [zit. b. (1)].

(9) COLTEN, H. R., L. P. EINSTEIN: Complement metabolism: Cellular and humoral regulation. Transplant. Rev. *32*: 3 (1976) [zit. b. (1)].

(10) HEREMANNS, J.: Les globulines seriques du système gamma. Edition Arscia S.A. Brucelles/ Masson et Cie., Paris 1960 [zit. b. (11)].

(11) JONAS, D., B. JÖVENER: Immunologische Serumproteinbestimmung im Exprimat bei chronischer Prostatitis. Med. Welt *24*: 872 (1973).

(12) LENNERT, K. A.: Immunologische Untersuchungen zur Pathogenese der chronischen Prostatitis. Urologe A *9*: 297 (1970).

(13) SELL, S.: Immunologie, Immunpathologie und Immunität, p. 270. Verlag Chemie, Weinheim—New York 1977.

(14) SOMER, T., D. J. WALLACE, P. T. FAN: Immune complex mediated rheumatic diseases. Ann. clin. Res. *12*: 77 (1980).

Institut für Medizinische Mikrobiologie, Zentrum für Dermatologie und Urologie
der Universität Gießen

Presence of Secretory- and Serum-IgA in Seminal Plasma

A. Sziegoleit, W. Krause, H.-C. Becker, W. Weidner

Introduction

Defence against infectious agents is related to the availability of specific immunoglobulins. Tomasi and Ziegelbaum have shown IgA to be the predominant immunoglobulin in secretory fluids and this class of immunoglobulins appears to assume importance with regard to infections arising at mucous membrane surfaces (Tomasi and Grey, 1962). Whereas serum IgA is present in monomer 7S form, the principle product of the mucosal plasma cell is a dimeric IgA molecule connected by a glycoprotein, the J chain. Another polypeptide, termed the secretory component, is synthesized in the mucosal epithelial cells where it is exposed on the basolateral cell surface as a specific receptor for dimeric IgA. After binding to the secretory component via disulfide bonding, the immunoglobulin complex is translocated through the epithelial cell (Nagura et al., 1979). The presence of secretory component on the IgA molecule thus indicates its origin from a mucosal tissue.

The aim of this study was to determine the presence of IgA in seminal plasma and to attempt a correlation between the appearance of "free" IgA with other parameters of acute inflammatory reactions within the urogenital tract.

Materials and methods

80 unselected semen specimens from patients suffering from andrological diseases were examined for the presence of bacteria and mycoplasmas, leucocytes, erythrocytes, IgA, IgG, C3 complement component and coeruloplasmin. The microbiological procedures were as described by Weidner et al. (1978), leucocytes and erythrocytes were counted in a cell counting chamber, proteins were quantitatively determined after centrifugation of the specimens ($12,000 \times g$, 2 min) by radial immunodiffusion (Tri-Partigen plates, Behringwerke AG, Marburg). The discrimination between serum IgA and secretory

IgA was performed by double diffusion analyses with α-chain-specific anti-serum (Behringwerke), with antiserum specific for secretory component (Dakopatts Immunoglobulins, Copenhagen, Denmark), and with an antiserum to IgA (Dakopatts) that precipitated IgA as well as secretory component.

Secretory IgA was isolated from human colostrum according to GROV, 1976.

Results

On the basis of the IgA analyses, three groups were distinguished. In the first group (n = 26), IgA consisted solely of secretory IgA; in a second group (n = 38), secretory IgA was accompanied by free secretory component; in the third group (n = 16), secretory IgA as well as serum IgA were detected. In the latter group, free secretory component was never found. Examples of the precipitation patterns obtained are depicted in Fig. 1.

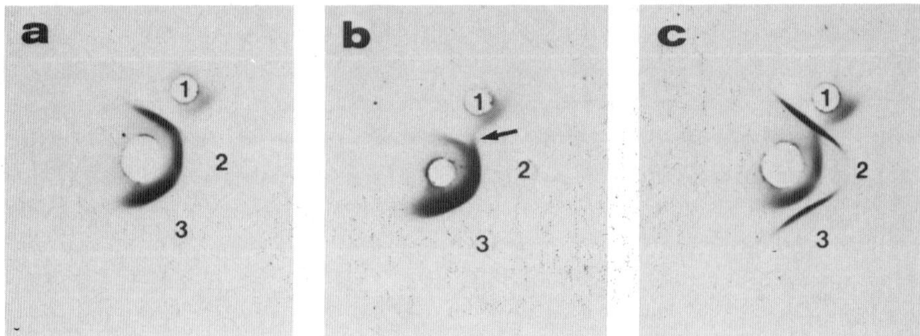

Fig. 1. Precipitation patterns of seminal plasma specimens (central wells) with antiserum against secretory component (1), α-chain specific antiserum (2) and antiserum against secretory IgA (3). *a:* illustrates a case where all detectable IgA is represented by secretory IgA. *b:* in this case, "free" (serum) IgA is additionally present (spur formation, arrow). *c:* illustrates a case where both secretory IgA and free secretory component are found. The small immunoprecipitates between wells 1 and 2 derive from IgA present in antiserum to secretory component (well 1).

Taking into consideration the other parameters tested (see Table 1), the third group of specimens (containing serum IgA) in all cases had significantly higher values of cell counts as well as of IgG, coeruloplasmin and C3. The occurrence of serum IgA in seminal fluids therefore may reflect a state of serum transsudation as occuring during acute inflammatory processes. The presence of free secretory component on the other hand was not accompanied by an increase of any other parameters tested. Regrettably, the microbiological

Table 1. Analysis of 80 semen specimens. Three groups were distinguished on the basis of their IgA composition. sIgA = secretory IgA, SC = free secretory component. The data represent the highest and lowest value of each parameter tested. Differences in the values in the group containing free IgA additional to secretory IgA to the values of the other groups in all cases are of high significance.

	sIgA (n = 26)	sIgA + SC (n = 38)	sIgA + IgA (n = 16)
IgA mg/dl	1.6 − 3.4	1.3 − 3	3.4 − 11.4
IgG mg/dl	7.6 − 15	6.6 − 10.7	13.4 − 23
Complement C3c mg/dl	0 − 1.9	0.5 − 1.6	1.5 − 2.7
Coeruloplasmin mg/dl	0 − 0.6	0 − 0.5	0.8 − 2.9
Leucocytes 10^6/ml	0 − 2	0 − 1.9	1.4 − 6.4
Erythrocytes 10^6/ml	0	0 − 0.2	0.2 − 2
Microbiological analysis	5× U. urealyticum	3× U. urealyticum 1× Enterococci	1× U. urealyticum 2× gram negative rods

data were too sparse to permit any conclusions to be drawn with regard to bacterial infections.

In contrast to intestinal and bronchial secretory fluids, secretory IgA does not seem to predominate in seminal plasma. By radial immunodiffusion, the concentration of IgG appears to be approximately thrice that of IgA. However, these values may be subject to artefacts if seminal fluid IgA were to exhibit precipitation behaviour deviating from that of serum IgA, e. g. due to restricted diffusion in the agarose gels because of size differences. Therefore, secretory IgA was isolated from human colostrum. The isolation procedure yielded secretory IgA with a purity exceeding 95%. In comparison of the protein concentration values obtained according to the Lowry procedure with those obtained by radial immunodiffusion using serum IgA as standard, the latter values were found to be three to four times too low. Thus, IgG and IgA seem to be present in equivalent concentrations in the seminal plasma.

Discussion

The presented data have demonstrated the presence of secretory IgA in seminal fluids and therefore shown that secretory IgA is produced in the organs involved in the production of seminal plasma. Besides secretory IgA, immunoglobulins of the IgG class were regularly found, whose origin is unknown at present.

Serum IgA was detectable only when blood cells, coeruloplasmin and C3 were raised significantly over normal values, supporting the assumption that the presence of free IgA in seminal fluids is an indicator of an exsudative process, such as is given in acute inflammation. The sparse data obtained from the bacterial cultures may indicate that apart from inflammation, local congestion may also contribute to such an event. These data differ from the results reported by Fowler et al. (1982), who did not detect differences in the relation of serum IgA to secretory IgA between samples from infected and uninfected patients. The discrepancy may be based on different techniques used to discriminate the two types of IgA.

In addition to secretory IgA, free secretory component was also found in nearly 50% of the specimens, often in abundant quantities. The presence of free secretory component has been reported in colostrum (Crago et al., 1979) and in urethral secretions (Burdon, 1971). This polypeptide is synthesized by the mucosal cells where it combines covalently with dimeric IgA. A surplus production may thus reflect a state of irritation of the mucosal cells.

References

(1) Burdon, D. W.: Immunoglobulins in normal human urine and urethral secretions. Immunol. *21*: 363−368 (1971).
(2) Crago, S. S., J. Mestecky: Secretory component: interactions with intracellular and surface immunoglobulins of human lymphoid cells. J. of Immunol. *122*: 906−911 (1979).
(3) Fowler, J. E., D. L. Kaiser, M. Mariano: Immunologic response of the prostate to bacteriuria and bacterial prostatitis. J. Urol. *128*: 158−164 (1982).
(4) Grov, A.: Human colostral IgA interacting with staphylococcal protein A. Acta path. microbiol. scand. (Sect. C) *84*: 71−72 (1976).
(5) Lowry, O. H., N. J. Rosebrough, A. L. Farr, R. J. Randall: Protein measurement with the Folin Phenol Reagent. J. Biol. Chem. *193*: 265−275 (1951).
(6) Nagura, H., P. K. Nakane, W. R. Brown: Translocation of dimeric IgA through neoplastic colon cells in vitro. J. Immunol. *123*: 2359−2368 (1979).
(7) Tomasi, T. B., S. D. Ziegelbaum: The selective occurrence of A globulins in certain body fluids. J. clin. Invest. *42*: 1552−1558 (1963).
(8) Tomasi, T. B., H. M. Grey: Structure and function of immunoglobulin A. Progr. Allergy *16*: 81−213 (1972).
(9) Weidner, W., H. Brunner, W. Krause, C. F. Rothauge: Zur Bedeutung von Ureaplasma urealyticum bei unspezifischer Prostata-Urethritis. Dtsch. med. Wschr. *11*: 465−470 (1978).

Institut für Medizinische Mikrobiologie; Urologische Klinik;
Institut für Hygiene und Infektionskrankheiten der Tiere, Arbeitsgruppe Zoonosen;
Klinik für Physikalische Medizin, Balneologie und Rheumatologie;
Justus-Liebig-Universität Gießen

Rheumatoid Factor-negative Arthritides and Urogenital Infections in Men*

H. G. SCHIEFER, W. WEIDNER, H. KRAUSS, U. GERHARDT, K. L. SCHMIDT

Introduction

Rheumatoid factor-negative (sero-negative) arthritides comprise 1. Reiter's syndrome, 2. ankylosing spondylitis (Morbus Strümpell−Marie−Bechterew), 3. sexually acquired reactive arthritis (SARA) (KEAT et al., 1980), and 4. reactive arthritis associated with infections elsewhere in the body (KNAPP et al., 1981).

A genetic predisposition is assumed to be essentially involved in the development of these diseases since histocompatibility antigen HLA B 27 is strongly associated with sero-negative arthritides (AHO et al., 1975; BREWERTON, 1976).

Rheumatoid factor-negative arthritis is frequently associated with infections of the male urogenital tract (OLHAGEN, 1975; ROMANUS, 1953). In Reiter's disease urethritis is a predominant symptom. In patients with ankylosing spondylitis, chronic prostatitis has often been detected (OLHAGEN, 1975; ROMANUS, 1953). In previous studies, however, the only criterion for the diagnosis of prostatitis had been the finding of high leucocyte numbers in prostatic fluid. No studies have been performed yet to identify the etiologic agents involved.

In this investigation we applied diagnostic procedures which we had recently established for the examination of patients suffering from urethritis and prostatitis (SCHIEFER et al., 1983, 1984; WEIDNER et al., 1978, 1980, 1982a, 1982b, 1983a, 1983b), for the urological and microbiological examinations of patients suffering from rheumatoid factor-negative arthritis.

---

* This contribution is a slightly modified version of a paper originally published in *"Zentralblatt für Bakteriologie"* (A) *255*: 511−517 (1983), and is printed by permission of G. Fischer Verlag, Stuttgart.

Methods

After anamnestic exploration of the patients, their genitalia were thoroughly examined by inspection and palpation.

The diagnosis of balanitis was established when the glans penis was inflamed and infiltrated. A swab was microbiologically examined for bacteria, mycoplasmas, and fungi.

Leading clinical symptom of urethritis was spontaneous urethral discharge. The microbiological analysis of urethral discharge and first voided urine (VB1) specimens included the isolation and quantitative determination of bacteria, fungi, mycoplasmas, and Chlamydia trachomatis, as detailed previously (SCHIEFER et al., 1983, 1984).

Patients without discharge, and patients suffering from symptoms of prostatitis, epididymitis, or urinary tract infection, were examined following a diagnostic scheme according to the "four-specimens-technique" (MEARES et al., 1968). As detailed previously (SCHIEFER et al., 1983, 1984), first voided urine (VB1), bladder urine (VB2), prostatic secretions (EPS) obtained by standardized prostatic massage, and urine after prostatic massage (VB3), were quantitatively analyzed for bacteria, fungi, and mycoplasmas. In addition EPS was cultivated for Neisseria gonorrhoeae and Chlamydia trachomatis. VB3 was microscopically examined for Trichomonas vaginalis. VB2 and VB3 samples were examined for polymorphonuclear leucocytes (PML): 3 ml each of VB2 and VB3 were cytocentrifuged, and the sedimented material was transferred to a slide and stained according to PAPANICOLAOU. In case of VB2 samples free of leucocytes (≤ 2), the total number of PML in VB3 was determined in five areas using a 400-fold magnification: ≤ 2 PML/microscopic field were regarded as normal, ≤ 4 PML as borderline value, and >4 PML as pathognomonic for prostatitis (WEIDNER et al., 1983a, 1983b).

Urethritis and prostatitis were classified according to previously published criteria (SCHIEFER et al., 1983, 1984).

In case of urinary tract infection, all urine specimens contained $>10^5$ cfu of common bacteria per ml.

Epididymitis was clinically diagnosed from the painfully infiltrated, swollen epididymis.

All microbiological studies were performed as previously described (BRUNNER et al., 1983; SCHIEFER et al., 1983, 1984; WEIDNER et al., 1978, 1980, 1982a, 1982b, 1983a, 1983b).

Results

146 men with rheumatoid factor − negative arthritis attended the special out-patient department for prostatitis. The arthritides were classified according to rheumatological criteria: 97 men suffered from ankylosing spondylitis, 36 from Reiter's syndrome, and 13 from reactive arthritis (Table 1).

Table 1. Rheumatoid factor-negative arthritis and urogenital tract infections.

	Total number of patients (n = 146)	Ankylosing Spondylitis (n = 97)	Reiter's Syndrome (n = 36)	Reactive Arthritis (n = 13)
No infection	72	60	6	6
Urogenital tract infection	74	37	30	7
Balanitis	3	–	3	–
Urethritis	14	–	13	1
Prostatitis	49	31	13	5
Epididymitis	1	1	–	–
Urinary tract infection	7	5	1	1

As further shown in Table 1, evidence for urogenital tract infections was obtained in 74 of 146 men (50.7%): 3 patients suffered from balanitis, 14 from urethritis, 49 from prostatitis, 1 from epididymitis, and 7 from urinary tract infection. Balanitis and urethritis were almost exclusively associated with Reiter's syndrome, whereas 31 of 37 men with ankylosing spondylitis and urogenital infection suffered from prostatitis.

In all cases (n = 3) with balanitis, enterococci were isolated.

In urethritis (n = 14), 2 patients suffered from gonorrhoea, and 12 from an infection with Chlamydia trachomatis. In 4 patients the chlamydial infection was combined with significantly high numbers of Ureaplasma urealyticum in urethral discharge ($\geq 10^4$ cfu/ml) and VB1 ($\geq 10^3$ cfu/ml).

In the one case with epididymitis, Chlamydia trachomatis was isolated from urethral swab after prostatic massage; additionally Ureaplasma urealyticum was isolated in significantly high numbers, i.e., similar to findings in prostatitis, $< 10^3$ cfu/ml VB1 and VB2, $\geq 10^4$ cfu/ml EPS, and $\geq 10^3$ cfu/ml VB3.

Urinary tract infections (n = 7) were caused by gram-negative bacteria and enterococci.

Table 2. Etiologic classification of prostatitis in patients suffering from rheumatoid factor-negative arthritis and prostatitis.

Etiologic agents isolated from patients with prostatitis	Total number of patients (n = 49)	Ankylosing Spondylitis (n = 31)	Reiter's Syndrome (n = 13)	Reactive Arthritis (n = 5)
Ureaplasma urealyticum	5	4	–	1
Chlamydia trachomatis	29	15	12	2
Escherichia coli	2	1	–	1
High leucocyte counts only* (no agent found)	13	11	1	1

* Prostatitis was diagnosed when, in the sediment of 3 ml of urine voided after prostatic massage
(VB3), >4 granulocytes were seen per microscopic field at 400-fold magnification.

As shown in Table 2, 31 of 97 patients (32%) with ankylosing spondylitis
suffered from prostatitis, as indicated by the finding of >4 PML per microscopic field at 400-fold magnification. In 4 men prostatitis was associated with
significantly high numbers of Ureaplasma urealyticum in typical prostatitis
constellation, i. e., $<10^3$ cfu/ml VB1 and VB2, $\geq 10^4$ cfu/ml EPS, and $\geq 10^3$ cfu/
ml VB3. In one man chronic bacterial prostatitis due to Escherichia coli was
diagnosed. In 15 men Chlamydia trachomatis was isolated from urethral swabs
or prostatic fluid after prostatic massage. In 11 patients no infectious agent
could be isolated.

Discussion

In 32% of patients suffering from ankylosing spondylitis, a prostatitis was
diagnosed by high leucocyte numbers in prostatic secretions. Our results correspond to observations of ROMANUS (1953) and KOHLIČEK and ŠVEC (1977).
As concerns the etiologic agents presumably involved, chronic bacterial and
ureaplasma-associated prostatitis is of minor importance. On the other hand,
the high isolation rate of Chlamydia trachomatis from EPS and/or urethral
swabs after standardized prostatic massage must be cautiously interpreted,
since we are well aware that the cultivated C. trachomatis might have originated from the urethra. Quantitative isolation studies similar to those in ureaplasmal diseases (BRUNNER et al., 1983; WEIDNER et al., 1978), and systematic
serological investigations (KRAUSS et al., 1983) have not been performed in
these cases. However, from other studies (KRAUSS et al., 1983; WEIDNER et al.,

1983 b) on "abacterial prostatitis" we have obtained good evidence that a correlation exists between cultivation of C. trachomatis as sole pathogen in cases of prostatitis, high leucocyte numbers in prostatic secretions, and detection of humoral antibodies against C. trachomatis by microimmunofluorescence test.

The pathogenesis of ankylosing spondylitis is still unclear. The molecular mimicry hypothesis (Ebringer, 1979, 1982) suggests that immunological cross-reactivity occurs between certain microorganisms and histocompatibility antigen HLA B 27 and might be responsible for development of ankylosing spondylitis. An infection of the prostate may be more directly involved, since antibodies against prostatic tissue were often detected in sera of patients with ankylosing spondylitis (Grimble, 1964). Until now the cause of prostatitis was assumed to be unknown (Kohliček et al., 1977). In our opinion the recently available data on Ureaplasma urealyticum (Brunner et al., 1983; Weidner et al., 1978) and Chlamydia trachomatis (Krauss et al., 1983; Schiefer et al., 1984; Weidner et al., 1983 b) infections of the prostate provide new aspects for the discussion of trigger mechanisms of rheumatic diseases by infectious prostatitis.

Acknowledgements

This work was supported by the Fraunhofer-Gesellschaft, München. Mrs. Lore Gottsmann provided excellent secretarial assistance.

References

(1) Aho, K., P. Ahvonen, P. Alkio, A. Lassus, E. Sairanen, K. Sievers, A. Tiilikainen: HLA 27 in reactive arthritis following infection. Ann. Rheum. Dis. *34* (Suppl. I): 29−30 (1975).

(2) Brewerton, D. A.: HLA − B 27 and the inheritance of susceptibility to rheumatic disease. Arthritis Rheum. *19*: 656−668 (1976).

(3) Brunner, H., W. Weidner, H. G. Schiefer: Studies on the role of Ureaplasma urealyticum and Mycoplasma hominis in prostatitis. J. Infect. Dis. *147*: 807−813 (1983).

(4) Ebringer, A.: Ankylosing spondylitis, immune response genes and molecular mimicry. Lancet *I*: 1186 (1979).

(5) Ebringer, A.: Spondylitis ankylosans und Klebsiellen: ein genetischer Zusammenhang? Münch. med. Wschr. *124*: 120−122 (1982).

(6) Grimble, A.: Auto-immunity to prostate antigen in rheumatic disease. J. Clin. Pathol. *17*: 264−267 (1964).

(7) Keat, A. C., B. J. Thomas, D. Taylor-Robinson, G. D. Pegrum, R. N. Maini, J. T. Scott: Evidence of Chlamydia trachomatis infection in sexually acquired reactive arthritis. Ann. Rheum. Dis. *39*: 431−437 (1980).

(8) Knapp, W., B. Prögel, C. Knapp: Immunpathologische Komplikationen bei enteralen Yersiniosen. Dtsch. med. Wschr. *106*: 1054−1060 (1981).

(9) Kohliček, J., V. Švec: Prostatitis chronica und Morbus Bechterew. Zschr. Urol. *70*: 827−831 (1977).

(10) KRAUSS, H., H. G. SCHIEFER, W. WEIDNER, M. ARENS, H. EBNER: Significance of Chlamydia trachomatis in "abacterial" prostatitis. Zbl. Bakt. A *254*: 545–551 (1983).

(11) MEARES, E. M., T. A. STAMEY: Bacteriologic localization patterns in bacterial prostatitis and urethritis. Invest. Urol. *5*: 492–518 (1968).

(12) OLHAGEN, B.: Chronic arthritis and prostatitis. In: DANIELSON, D., L. JUHLIN, P.-A. MÅRDH (eds.): Clinical pattern and therapy: genital infections and their complications; pp. 211–214. Almqvist and Wiksell, Stockholm 1975.

(13) ROMANUS, R.: Pelveospondylitis ossificans in the male and genitourinary infection. Acta Med. Scand. (Suppl.) *280*: 1–368 (1953).

(14) SCHIEFER, H. G., W. WEIDNER, H. KRAUSS, U. GERHARDT, K. L. SCHMIDT: Rheumatoid factor – negative arthritis, especially ankylosing spondylitis, and infections of the male urogenital tract. Zbl. Bakt. A *255*: 511–517 (1983).

(15) SCHIEFER, H. G., W. WEIDNER, H. KRAUSS, U. GERHARDT, W. KRAUSE: Prostatitis as sequela of non-gonococcal urethritis – a prospective study. In: BRUNNER, H., W. KRAUSE, C. F. ROTHAUGE, W. WEIDNER (eds.): Chronic Prostatitis; pp. 75–83. Schattauer, Stuttgart–New York 1984.

(16) WEIDNER, W., H. BRUNNER, W. KRAUSE, C. F. ROTHAUGE: Zur Bedeutung von Ureaplasma urealyticum bei unspezifischer Prostato-Urethritis. Dtsch. med. Wschr. *103*: 465–470 (1978).

(17) WEIDNER, W., H. G. SCHIEFER, H. KRAUSS, J. ENGSTFELD: Chlamydia trachomatis und Ureaplasma urealyticum bei unspezifischer Urethritis. Helv. Chir. Acta *47*: 417–421 (1980).

(18) WEIDNER, W., H. G. SCHIEFER, H. KRAUSS, J. ENGSTFELD: Untersuchungen zur Ätiologie der nicht-gonorrhoischen Urethritis. Dtsch. med. Wschr. *107*: 1227–1231 (1982a).

(19) WEIDNER, W., H. G. SCHIEFER, K. L. SCHMIDT: Urogenitale Infektionen bei seronegativer "reaktiver" Arthritis und ankylosierender Spondylitis. Akt. Rheumatol. *7*: 82–85 (1982b).

(20) WEIDNER, W., H. EBNER: Zytologische Analyse des Exprimaturins – eine Möglichkeit zur Klassifikation der Prostatitis? In: BRUNNER, H., W. KRAUSE, C. F. ROTHAUGE, W. WEIDNER (eds.): Chronische Prostatitis; pp. 173–182. Schattauer, Stuttgart–New York 1983a.

(21) WEIDNER, W., M. ARENS, H. KRAUSS, H. G. SCHIEFER, H. EBNER: Chlamydia trachomatis in "abacterial" prostatitis: microbiological, cytological and serological studies. Urol. int. *38*: 146–149 (1983b).

Dermatologische Klinik und Poliklinik der Universität München
(Direktor: Prof. Dr. Dr. h. c. O. Braun-Falco)
Abteilung für klinische Chemie und klinische Biochemie (Direktor: Prof. Dr. H. Fritz)
an der Chirurgischen Klinik der Universität München
Urologische Abteilung des Städt. Krankenhauses Thalkirchner Straße, München
(Direktor: Prof. Dr. A. Hofstetter)

Proteinases and Proteinase Inhibitors in Ejaculates of Men with Adnex Affections

M. Jochum, W.-B. Schill, E. Fink, A. Friesen, A. Hofstetter, H. Schiessler

Introduction

Proteinases of the male genital tract are important primarily for the fertilization process. They are taking part also in coagulation and liquefaction of ejaculate as well as in stimulation of sperm migration within the female genital secretions. Moreover, proteinases are involved as mediators of the inflammatory response in the male genital tract aggravating the clinical symptoms (Schill, 1975; Hafez, 1976; Havemann and Janoff, 1978).

These proteinases are either sperm specific enzymes (acrosin), secretory products of the accessory sexual glands (seminin, BAEE-splitting enzyme, urokinase, tissue kallikrein) or they are liberated in the adnexal region during degranulation of leukocytes (elastase).

In the male genital tract proteolytic activity of the proteinases are kept under control by potent antagonists, the high molecular weight plasma proteinase inhibitors α_1-proteinase inhibitor (formally α_1-antitrypsin) and α_1-antichymotrypsin as well as the low molecular weight, acid-stable secretory products leukostatin (HUSI-I) and acrostatin (HUSI-II) (Schiessler et al., 1976; Schill, 1976; Schiessler and Schill, 1977; Schill and Schiessler, 1977).

We were interested, therefore, to see whether in chronic adnex affections alterations in the proteinase/proteinase inhibitor system of the ejaculate are measurable, probably qualified as diagnostic criteria.

Material and methods

Ejaculates were withdrawn from patients undergoing standard diagnostics such as 3-tube test and analysis of the urethral smear, prostatic fluid and urine. Diagnosis of chronic adnexitis was confirmed by the following criteria: significantly high numbers of gram-negative bacteria, enterococci, mycoplasmas, Ureaplasma urealyticum and Chlamydia trachomatis, leukocytes more than 20 per visual field; evidence of complement factor 3c and coeruloplasmin in seminal plasma. Ejaculates from 40 patients with adnex affections were examinated; 14 patients showed vegetative urogenital syndrome (VUG) and anogenital symptomcomplex (AGS), 24 patients suffered from chronic and 2 from acute adnexitis. Within the group of chronic adnexitis patients were further differenciated according to the concentration of the complement factor 3c as follows: patients with C3c values lower (n = 14) or higher (n = 10) than 1.2 mg%, respectively. Activities of seminin, urokinase, and the BAEE-splitting enzyme in seminal plasma were determined using known methods (FRITZ, 1972; SCHILL, 1973). Tissue kallikrein was quantified by a specific radioimmunoassay (FINK and GÜTTL, 1978). The immunological concentrations of α_1-proteinase inhibitor, α_1-antichymotrypsin, acrostatin and leukostatin were measured by radial immunodiffusion ("Mancini-technique"). The concentration of liberated granulocytic elastase bound to α_1-proteinase inhibitor (E-α_1PI) was estimated by a newly developed enzyme-linked immunoassay (NEUMANN et al., 1983). Statistical evaluation was performed by the independent Student-t-test.

Results and discussion

Significance and physiological function of the BAEE-splitting enzyme from prostatic secretions is rather unknown. So far, only during viscosity disturbances of seminal plasma, a clearly lowered enzyme activity could be proven (SCHILL, personal communication). Seminin, originating also from prostata, is involved in clotting and liquefaction of sperm. Moreover, it may facilitate penetration of spermatozoa into cervix mucus. In contrast to normal ejaculates, both enzymes showed a significant decrease during chronic adnexitis as well in VUG as in AGS. This might be caused probably by massage of prostata before ejaculation. With acute adnexitis, a clear increase in enzyme-concentrations was measurable in accordance with a commonly observed enhancement of organ function and synthesis during acute inflammatory reactions (Fig. 1).

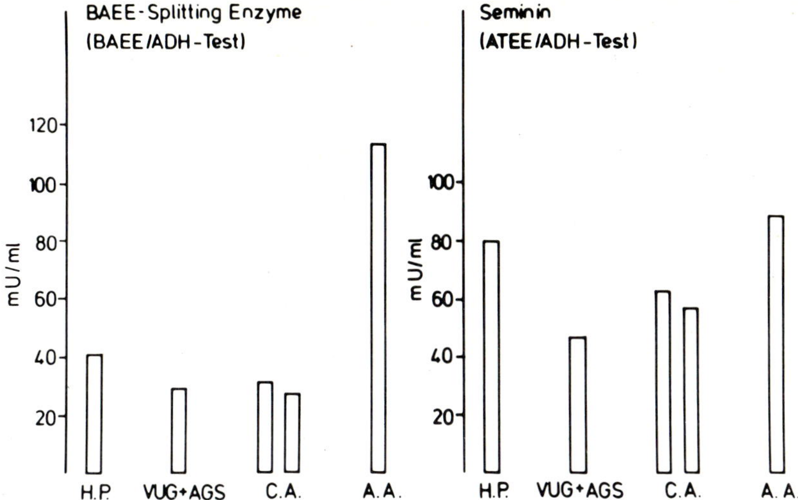

Fig. 1. Activity of BAEE-splitting enzyme and seminin in ejaculates of men with adnex affections (H. P. = healthy persons; VUG = vegetative urogenital syndrome; AGS = anogenital symptom complex; C. A. = chronic adnexitis with complement factor C3 <1.2 mg% or >1.2 mg%, respectively; A. A. = acute adnexitis).

Urokinase and tissue kallikrein were also demonstrable in prostatic secretion; their physiological relevance, however, ist still unknown. Probably, tissue kallikrein takes part in stimulation and maintenance of spermatozoon motility via liberation of pharmacologically highly active kinins from sperm plasma kininogen. In comparison to healthy persons, both enzymes showed a slight, though statistically not significant reduction in patients with chronic adnexitis and VUG; again, in acute adnexitis an expected increase of the enzymes' concentrations was measurable (Fig. 2).

The high molecular weight plasma proteinase inhibitors α_1-proteinase inhibitor and α_1-antichymotrypsin, transudated from serum into seminal plasma, showed no significant alterations during VUG, AGS or chronic adnexitis, respectively. However, throughout acute adnexitis the well-known dramatic increase of the inhibitors' concentrations was demonstrable in seminal plasma. This enhancement may be due not only to a considerably increased synthesis of the inhibitors as acute phase proteins during the acute inflammatory response but also to a lowered blood-seminal plasma-barrier (Fig. 3).

The acid-stable, low molecular weight proteinase inhibitor leukostatin synthesized in the vesicular glands is supposed to be the natural antagonist of leukocyte proteinases. It did not exhibit significant alterations. The same holds true for acrostatin (Fig. 4), the highly potent inhibitor of the penetration enzyme acrosin which is localized in the acrosome of the spermatozoon. The low

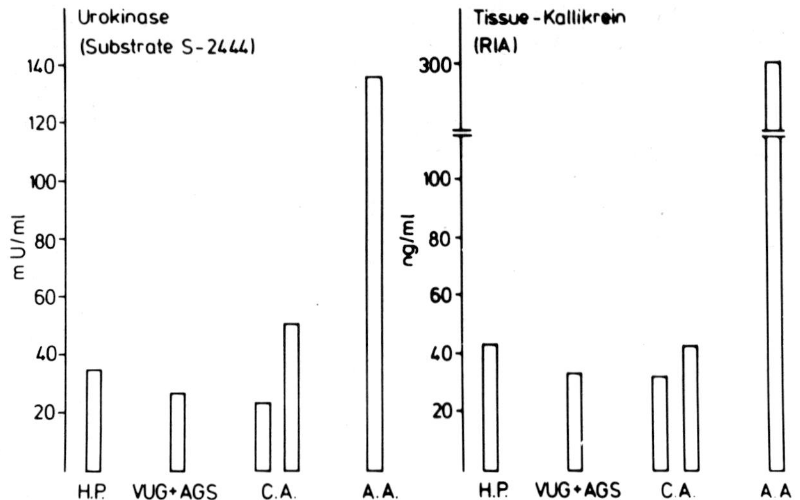

Fig. 2. Activity of urokinase and concentration of tissue kallikrein in ejaculates of men with adnex affections.

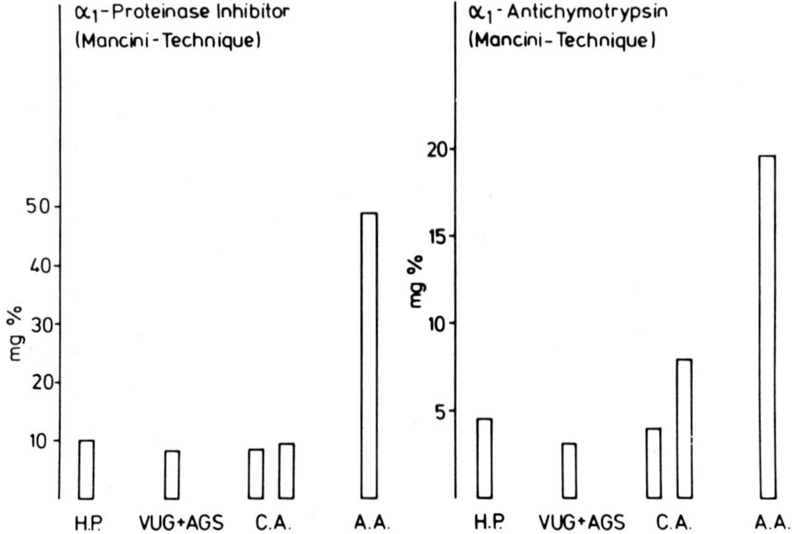

Fig. 3. Concentrations of α_1-proteinase inhibitor and a_1-antichymotrypsin in ejaculates of men with adnex affections.

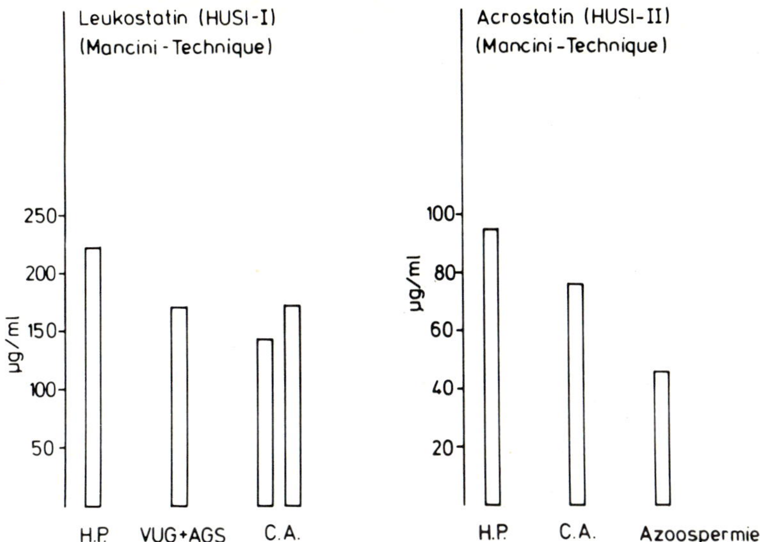

Fig. 4. Concentrations of leukostatin and acrostatin in ejaculates of men with adnex affections.

molecular weight, acid-stable acrostatin — synthesized in vesicular glands and epididymis — showed a clear reduction of the inhibitor concentration only in man with occlusive azoospermia (SCHILL and SCHIESSLER, 1977).

Summarizing the given data, the proteinases and proteinase inhibitors described above did not turn out to be significant diagnostic parameters in chronic adnexitis, VUG and AGS, respectively. This is, however, different with leukocytic proteinases during these inflammatory processes.

The biological function of leukocytic proteinases is the intracellular protein catabolism of wasted endogenous substances and the degradation of phagocytized invasive organisms. If released extracellularly due to degranulation or disintegration of leukocytes, these proteinases may enhance tissue damage and activation of the inflammatory response. Of the leukocytic proteinases known so far, the neutral proteinase elastase from polymorphonuclear granulocytes deserves special interest because of its high amount within the granules as well as its nearly unlimited cleavage specificity. However, due to a relatively rapid reaction with α_1-proteinase inhibitor, the most important inhibitor of this enzyme, granulocytic elastase liberated extracellularly is found nearly exclusively in an already inactivated form.

With a highly sensitive enzyme-linked immunoassay about 180 ng complexed elastase (E-α_1-PI) per ml were found in ejaculates of 10 healthy persons. Patients with VUG and AGS showed a highly significant elevation up to x =

1100 ng/ml. In chronic adnexitis a similar increase (x = 1200 ng/ml) could be shown in seminal plasma containing C3c concentrations below 1.2 mg%, whereas C3 amounts above 1.2 mg% were combined with a further dramatic increase of complexed elastase up to 4500 ng/ml. Moreover, in acute adnexitis elastase levels far more than 10,000 ng/ml were measured (Fig. 5).

From these preliminary results of 40 ejaculates, which of course will be confirmed with a more extended patient collective, we draw the following conclusions:

1. The levels of complexed granulocytic elastase proved to be a highly sensitive and qualified parameter of inflammatory processes in adnex affections.

2. Most of the biochemical parameters determined so far in ejaculates of patients with adnex affections are only an indirect criterion of an impaired blood-seminal plasma-barrier during the inflammatory process. Levels of complexed granulocytic elastase, however, represent a direct quantification of an inflammatory mediator in the adnexial region.

3. Quantification of complexed elastase might become a reliable biochemical parameter additional to diagnostic criteria used now in adnex affections. This new parameter seems to reflect activity and severity of an inflammatory process more specifically and offers, therefore, new aspects for controlling the course of the disease as well as the therapy.

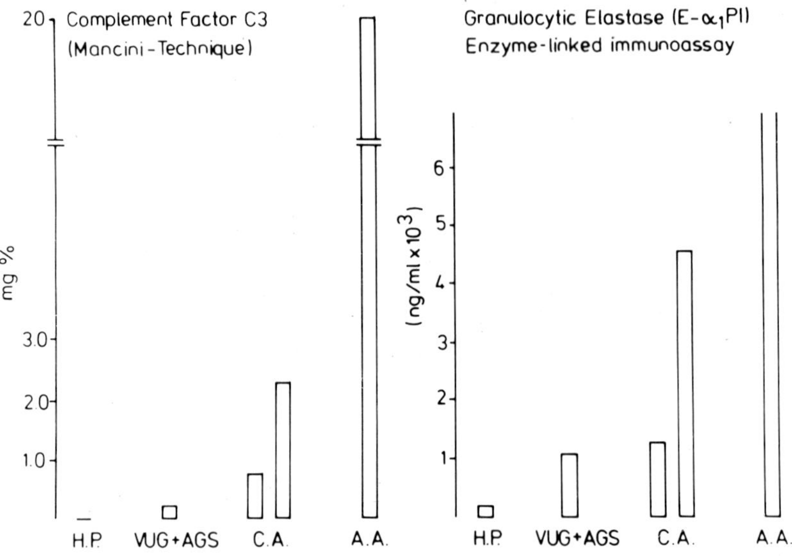

Fig. 5. Concentrations of complement factor 3c and granulocytic elastase in complex with α_1-proteinase inhibitor (E-α_1PI) in ejaculates of men with adnex affections.

References

(1) FINK, E., C. GÜTTL: Development of a radioimmunoassay for pig pancreatic kallikrein. J. Clin. Chem. Clin. Biochem. *16*: 381−385 (1978).

(2) FRITZ, H., M. ARNHOLD, B. FÖRG-BREY, L. J. D. ZANEVELD, G. F. B. SCHUMACHER: Verhalten der "Chymotrypsinähnlichen" Proteinase aus Humansperma gegenüber Protein-Proteinase-Inhibitoren. Hoppe-Seyler's Z. Physiol. Chem. *353*: 1651−1653 (1972).

(3) HAFEZ, E. S. E. (ed.): Human Semen and Fertility Regulation in Men. Mosby, St. Louis 1976.

(4) HAVEMANN, K., A. JANOFF (eds.): Neutral Proteases of Human Polymorphonuclear Leukocytes. Urban & Schwarzenberg, Baltimore−Munich 1978.

(5) NEUMANN, S., N. HENNRICH, G. GUNZER, H. LANG: Enzymelinked Immunoassay for complexes of Human Elastase with α_1-Proteinase Inhibitor in Plasma. In: GOLDBERG, D. M., M. WERNER (eds.): Progress in Clinical Enzymology II, Masson Publ., New York 1983.

(6) SCHIESSLER, H., M. ARNHOLD, K. OHLSSON, H. FRITZ: Inhibitors of Acrosin and Granulocytes Proteinases from Human Genital Tract Secretions. Hoppe-Seyler's Z. Physiol. Chem. *357*: 1251−1260 (1976).

(7) SCHIESSLER, H., W.-B. SCHILL: Proteinaseinhibitoren in menschlichem Sperma: Biochemie und Biologische Funktion. Fortschr. d. Fertilitätsforschung 5: 189−191 (1977).

(8) SCHILL, W.-B.: Akrosin Activity in Human Spermatozoa: Methodological Investigations. Arch. Derm. Forsch. *248*: 257−273 (1973).

(9) SCHILL, W.-B.: Quantitative Determination of High Molecular Weight Serum Proteinase Inhibitors in Human Semen. Andrologia 8: 359−364 (1976).

(10) SCHILL, W.-B.: Die Bedeutung proteolytischer Spermaenzyme für die Fertilität. Hautarzt 26: 514−523 (1975).

(11) SCHILL, W.-B., H. SCHIESSLER: Proteinaseinhibitoren in menschlichem Sperma: Quantitative Bestimmung und klinische Aspekte. Fortschritte der Fertilitätsforschung 5: 192−194 (1977).

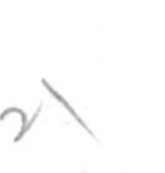